Why Can't You Just Behave?

Why Can't You Just Behave?

Uncovering Your Child
Masked Behind *Bad* Behaviors

BRITTA HELAYNE

Why Can't You Just Behave?

ISBN 978-0-578-60178-6

Printed in The United States of America

Cover Assistance by Alexander Kliafas

Cover Photo by Jensen Morgan

General Assistance by Cameron Morgan

This book is dedicated to

My Mom, who gave me the time to write,

My oldest son Cameron, who showed me the tools to write,

My second son Jensen, who taught me to be a better writer,

My twin son Benji, who encouraged me to keep going,

My twin son Braeden, who is my inspiration and my story.

Without them, I would have never had the opportunity to go on this journey.

CONTENTS

SECTION 1 BEHAVIORS ARE MORE THAN A SET OF ACTIONS

SECTION 2 THE WHOLE CHILD

SECTION 3 PARENTING THE WHOLE CHILD PROGRAM

APPENDIX

INTRODUCTION

Welcome! I'm so glad you are reading this book! My name is Britta, and I once stood in your shoes. I know what it is like to look for answers dealing with your child's bad behavior but never really finding a solution that works. I have had the sleepless nights wondering what the next day would bring for my out of control child. I have worried about how I was going to handle or get through one more day of exhaustion because of my child's bad behavior. I have felt shame and guilt about the reflection of my parenting because of the misbehavior of my child. I have also felt the overwhelming sense of relief when I found answers to help my child overcome negativity and thrive. It is time for bad behavior to stop controlling your child and your family's life. All of that can change for you, and I will show you how. If you are an overwhelmed, stressed-out parent looking for answers, this is for you. If you are a parent or caregiver that struggles with a child, this is for you. If you are a parent that has looked for answers but feels lost, this is for you. If you want to prevent bad behaviors in your child, this is for you too!

Regardless of why you are here, I am so glad you made it.

In this book, I offer practical, easy to follow instructions about how to transform where you are now to a lifestyle that is less complicated by bad behaviors. This book is straight forward and can get your family

1

healthy in a shorter amount of time because we will deal with the root of bad behavior, not just treat and deal with the actions alone. The journey is not an easy one; however, I promise it is easier than dealing with a child that continually has bad behaviors. Follow me on this journey, stick with the steps in this book, and I promise you will be grateful for the time you invested in yourself and your child.

There are a few tips I'd like to share with you before you get started reading. This book has 3 Sections. The first Section is my story, the second is an overview of different aspects of health, and the third and final Section is a plan of action steps to create a transformation of bad behavior to balanced healthy behavior. It is best to follow each Section in order. After each Chapter, I have listed Journaling Points and a Final Thought. To get the most out of this book, use a journal, a binder with loose paper works best, and write your answers to the Journaling Points as you read through each Chapter. In Section 3, a journal is a must for the transformation stage. Starting a journal from the beginning will help you navigate through Section 3 quicker.

Lastly, I would love to hear your answers to the questions I have asked, if you are willing to share. I have been on the same journey you are about to undergo, but I didn't have a blueprint like I have laid out for you to follow. I hope to help you navigate through parenting bad behaviors, so your child and family can live peaceful and healthy lives. Please reach out to me on Facebook,

Instagram, or my website and share your struggles as I have shared with you!

I look FORWARD to hearing from you!

SECTION 1

BEHAVIORS ARE MORE THAN A SET OF ACTIONS

CHAPTER 1

BRAEDEN'S STORY

"Either he's moving out of the house, or I'm moving out, but we both cannot stay," those words actually came to my mind when one of my twin boys pushed me to the limit, and I was at the end of trying. I had tried everything with Braeden, all but four years old at the time, to behave. Nothing worked. Nothing! Not the multiple discipline and parenting books I read, not the reward charts or speaking positively, not even a treasure chest or special alone time. The pediatrician's advice didn't work, the information I found online, or suggestions from older wiser moms whose kids seemed to be ultra-perfect compared to mine. I was failing and failing fast. As this child became older, I became less qualified to discipline and take care of him. As a mother of four boys, Braeden being the youngest, a twin beat by his older twin by a whole seven minutes, I felt like the worst parent because I could not get this child under control. His behavior affected the entire family and how I viewed myself as an effective mom. I was overwhelmed with guilt and felt I was just not a good enough parent.

Really, Braeden had more going on than bad behaviors. He had other problems with his health as well, starting right when he was born. Braeden and his twin Benji were born at 34 weeks. Braeden was the weaker of the two and was placed on a breathing machine immediately after he was delivered. Both were put in ICU, although Benji was mostly keeping his twin company. In the first few years of his life, Braeden had multiple health issues that required frequent trips to the doctor. He had acid reflux that was supposed to go away after he learned to sit but didn't until well into his second year of life. He continually had horrible bouts of croup that none of his other brothers ever seemed to get. Braeden required regular breathing treatments on a nebulizer starting when he was nine months old. He had chronic conditions of ear infections, eczema, and rosy red cheeks and ears. Braeden drooled so badly he had to wear a bib all the time or have his shirt frequently changed, which is typical for a baby, but for him, it was up until the age of four.

As Braeden grew, the problems worsened and became bigger problems, physically and behaviorally. Getting Braeden to bed at night was a chore. As soon I left his room, like clockwork, he'd pop back up over and over. He frequently awoke at night for 20-30 minutes, uncontrollably crying and screaming for no apparent reason and the next morning remembering nothing. Then there were a few nights when he awoke gasping for air, needing to be rushed to the hospital. On occasion, he would even sleepwalk, which was scary because his room was on the second floor.

The bad behavior really started to take root after Braeden turned 3. He was a negative child, which was so odd to me, as I definitely lean more towards being positive, maybe even annoyingly so! He seemed to hate everything, and everything was a no. Braeden was almost happy when he saw negative things happen, smirking. He laughed many times when I was disciplining him or sent him for a time out. If I sent him to his room, really a time out for his brothers and I, he would throw things, open and slam the door shut repeatedly, or lay and kick his feet on the wall. Really? A child, this young, could be capable of this destructive behavior? He hit, kicked, bit, pushed, pulled on his brothers, or me on a regular basis. Braeden would walk by and destroy something and seemed to have no cares about what he just demolished. And then...there were...the tantrums. He had frequent outbursts several times a day. He had so many, I dreaded going out with him, in case I couldn't control or diffuse a situation that was likely to occur. These behaviors happened day after day, with nothing seeming to work. Everything just kept getting worse. I felt like I was stuck in a tunnel with no end in sight. What was I doing wrong?

You are never given more than you can handle. I had believed that statement. However, if that were true, why was I in this situation? It sure seemed to be more than I could handle! I was a mother of 4 precious boys I adored, loved, and would do anything for. My other boys were not perfect. However, they were not this constant tornado of bad behavior like this child, not even close. They didn't compare. I knew something was not right with Braeden, and it was apparent that focusing on his behavior was not working. No one was able to give me any answers to all the problems I was having with Braeden. So, what did that leave me? Was I the problem, or was it him? Did I need to take him to a specialized doctor for testing? Did he need to be medicated for his behaviors? And what would that mean for him...what would his diagnoses be? Braeden and Benji were approaching their first year of elementary school, all-day kindergarten, in just a few short months. It was the beginning of that summer that I decided I needed to do something and do it fast. It was time to think outside the box.

Does any of this sound familiar? Are you struggling right now with a child that has bad behaviors? Do you have a child that you know something isn't right, but you can't put your finger on what it is? Are you having a hard time getting answers from health professionals? Well, you are certainly not alone. I went through years of beating myself up, feeling responsible, and guilty about my child's behavior with no answers. It wasn't until I realized that behaviors are affected by more than actions, that everything started to turn around. I went from having a child that people didn't want to be around, to a transformed child still to this day astonishes and continually amazes me with his compassion and kindness. What I found, gave Braeden his personality back, something I didn't know even existed! I am on a mission to help other parents realize that they are, in fact, not bad parents, but it's time to parent in a different way.

Unlike mainstream parenting books, this book looks at and addresses the child as a whole. It does not simply suggest solutions to help with symptoms of your child's behavior. This book will dig deeper into the root causes of behavior. This book will discuss food and how it affects the brain, emotions, and functioning of the body. What role exercise has on the body will be addressed and which activities are best for your child. We will also look at how much sleep your child should be getting and what affects the quality of sleep. Meditation is also essential, and we will discuss how and why it can make a big difference in your child's life. Lastly, we will look at other influences, such as how your child thinks and talks to themselves and the environment. If you follow the steps in the book, not only will your child's life change, but the whole dynamics of your family's life will transform for the better. You will be able to help set your child on a path to success, a path that will start him or her off at any age and stay with them as adults. You can help your child form positive habits from the beginning that will last their entire life. Let's set your child up for success.

Journal Points

What has been the hardest part of dealing with your child's bad behaviors?

In what ways have you tried to change your parenting style to fix your child's bad behaviors?

Final Thought

You are not a bad parent. Your child is not a bad child. YOU can and will overcome this and I will help you!

CHAPTER 2

MY STORY

In November of 2007, I had a health crisis of my own. I was suffering from many symptoms such as loss of focus and concentration, allergies, sensitivities to many foods, extreme fatigue, and low blood sugar, to name a few. I went from one doctor, who sent me to another doctor, who sent me to another doctor and so on. Gradually, I noticed that when I ate certain foods, my symptoms became worse. I started to experiment with food and altered what I was eating. I kept a journal to link which foods were troublesome and which foods made me feel alive. Realizing what foods bothered my energy levels, moods, and physical symptoms, I decided to apply the same principles to Braeden, and this is when everything drastically transformed. It hurts my heart to think of that little boy with such bad behavior. After we changed to a healthier lifestyle, he dramatically changed. He was buried in symptoms, as I was, modifying his true personality.

I had no idea how much food affected the body until I felt the difference. Of course, I knew about the body needing vitamins and minerals to function correctly, that's why I bought fortified juices and cereals and took a multivitamin. That should cover everything, right?! Never mind, I was overweight and had continual sinus infections, despite having two sinus surgeries to correct any deficiencies. No one told me about food creating physical symptoms or affecting moods or energy levels in the body. I had never heard or read anything about that. It wasn't until the health crisis that I noticed foods making me feel worse than I already felt. I needed to be at the top of my game. I had four young children counting on me! I didn't want anything making me feel worse than I already felt.

Sugar was the first thing that I eliminated out of my diet. I noticed when I ate anything with sugar, I started to drag and feel lethargic, especially in the afternoon. Cutting sugar made my energy reserves skyrocket. I had more energy than I had ever remembered having. After sugar, I cut dairy, and suddenly all my sinus problems disappeared. I stopped taking medications that I had been on for years for my allergies. However, they didn't work as well as they once used to anyway.

Dairy was harder for me to take out of my diet. Back then, the alternatives were not as vast as they are these days. I missed eating cheese! But boy, if I cheated, I paid the price. I became congested and stuffy and even felt my mood change. A wave of sadness, just feeling down and not feeling like myself, came over me. I would think, "What's wrong with you? Why are you so unhappy? Nothing has changed. Where is this coming from?" It wasn't until I learned how food could affect your mood that I realized dairy could alter me so drastically! That was the end of cheating for me. I didn't need to eat anything that literally depressed me.

Since discovering food had such a profound effect on me, I dove into learning more about it and the chemical reactions in the body. I learned that food is medicine and should be treated with care. Whatever I ate would either strengthen me or weaken me, and weak was unacceptable. It was at this point I had an epiphany! I wondered if food made such a huge difference in my body, what was it doing to my children? What about Braeden? Could different foods improve his behavior? It was certainly worth a shot! It was time to do some experimenting.

I decided to implement some changes in both Braeden and his twin Benji's diet. Although Benji didn't have all the misbehaviors that Braeden had, he did have physical issues, such as chronic eczema, ear, and sinus infections. At the age of 4, Benji had his tonsils removed, and Braeden was up next to have his removed. Knowing that replacing dairy products helped me with my allergies and congestion, it was the first place I started in Braeden and Benji's diet. After all, it wouldn't hurt to replace the dairy for a short time to see what would happen. I could always bring it back to their diet. What would it hurt if the removal of dairy helped with the chronic conditions, they both experienced? Needless to say, Braeden never needed to get his tonsils out. He still has them to this day!

Within a short amount of time, I noticed small changes in both of them. Braeden's croup symptoms disappeared along with the need for nebulizer treatments. Eczema subsided, along with Benji's. Braeden's rosy red cheeks and ears turned back to a normal color. These results were astonishing! I couldn't believe the enormous impact cutting dairy had on both boys. I was shocked! Realizing dairy was hurting them, the Mommy guilt washed over me. I felt as though I was poisoning my boys from a very young age. Oh, how I pushed cheese, yogurts, and milk on the boys. I wanted them to grow properly, and I was taught dairy was a must to have strong bones.

Although most of Braeden's physical symptoms had disappeared with the removal of dairy, his behavior was nowhere near the improvement levels I was hoping to see. The leftover behavior still included night terrors and sleepwalking, the excess drooling, and all the naughtiness I explained before. I was ready to up my game and dig in to see what else I could do to help Braeden in this newfound way with food!

Eventually that summer, I did discover how a particular food, corn, could play a mastermind role in Braeden's behavior. I went on to eliminate corn out of his diet, which at the time seemed impossible! But what ended up being tough was dealing with the consequences of Braeden having corn. Corn was EASY to avoid compared to what it turned him into if he ate it. Eliminating corn meant saying goodbye to the drooling, the night issues, the destruction, pushing, hitting, biting, and the constant tantrums. A new child emerged; one I only saw very little of. A child that cared, shared and loved, and had a heart that was bigger than him. He was sensitive and placed others before him. He stopped saying no and hating what seemed like everything. I was blown away. I was relieved. I was bursting to let everyone know what I had at once knew nothing about, that each child is different and what can nourish one child can poison another.

With all these new things I was learning, I felt like a veil lifted from my eyes, and for the first time, I saw clearly. I became almost obsessed with learning about the body and what else had a significant effect like food had on it. All these different categories needed to be paid attention to for the body to function the way it is intended to. I saw how much I was doing not only to myself but to my children as well, that was going AGAINST what the individual body needed. I had the definition of parenting all wrong. I looked at parenting as managing and trying to shape behavior. I needed to teach my children how to be well-behaved kids WHILE nourishing them. I had hoped and wanted my kids to eat properly, but before my discovery, I had the wrong idea of what a proper diet and nourishment meant. I decided it was time to make a drastic lifestyle change. My children deserved to know how to take care of themselves and to feel as good as they could! They had no idea how good they could feel, how healthy they could become.

Everything turned around with Braeden. The moods, the bad behavior, the destruction all of it was gone. Now, of course, he wasn't a perfectly behaved little boy, he still had time outs and his moments. But the moments were not as constant as they used to be. We didn't need to hold our breath any longer with him. We could all just breathe. As I write this book, Braeden is now 15. I'm pretty sure if I told that story to his teachers or adults that know him, they would be surprised. Braeden is THE kindest, most compassionate kid. He would give you the shirt off his back. He's thoughtful, concerned about others, and can't stand to see people go without. It's like he was trapped in another body before we made a lifestyle change.

Looking back on the situation, knowing what I know now, I can see I was most likely dealing with a child that has ADHD and would have probably been medicated. I can't imagine not finding the answers I have discovered and having to still deal with all the behaviors throughout the years. I still see Braeden's brain working in ways that align with ADD/ADHD. However, we have the tools to be able to help him. See, Braeden had an underlying problem, and the foods I was feeding him magnified it. Now, he is equipped with what he needs to function and be himself without having to worry about what will influence his behavior and set physical and behavioral reactions off. It was a lifestyle change, and it was SO worth it. It is tough to struggle and watch a child with bad behaviors that you have no control over. It is much easier to feed a child with the right foods for their body and deal with any leftover problems. The leftover problems seem so insignificant compared to what we were dealing with before.

Is this book only going to help children with ADD/ADHD? Absolutely not. The point is, it doesn't matter the age, or if you have a diagnosis, it matters that you give the body what it needs for the individual. We either help the body or hurt it. It's easier to be proactive than to deal with a plethora of reactions.

In Section 2 of this book, I will introduce you to the different aspects of health and why they are essential. In Section 3, I will walk you through a 4 Step program to help you achieve real results for your child. If you are ready to stop parenting the symptoms and start parenting the whole child, stick with me, and I will walk with you every step of the way. Together, we will uncover your child that is masked behind bad behaviors.

Journal Points

How do you deal with the stress of your child's misbehaviors?

How would a transformation, like Braeden went through, change your life?

Final Thought

By the end of this book, you can have a success story, just like mine.

CHAPTER 3

WHAT CAN WE DO?

LOOKING BACK TO MOVE FORWARD

My ancestors moved to the United States in the late 1880s from Sweden and settled in the Midwest. They arrived in this country with very few possessions, but they had plenty of hopes, dreams, and plans for the future. My grandmother was a child of one of those direct descendants and is still living today at the age of 92. Grandma Lu loves to share snapshots of her life growing up in the Midwest farm country of rural Iowa. Her family lived in an average home, in an ordinary town. Her home life consisted of the standard nuclear family, including a mom, dad, and two children, a boy and a girl. Back then, it wasn't unusual to have an elder living with the parents, and Grandma Lu's family was no exception. Her grandmother lived with her family until she passed away in the 1930s.

Grandma Lu recalls having good fun, innocent memories of childhood. Memories of children playing outside from morning until night, the world being their playground. The neighbors would all watch out for each other's children, and if a child was up to no good, you could bet it got back to the parent from another adult in the town. In my Grandma Lu's case, the word always got back to her mom that she was out picking up dead birds and putting them in her little red wagon again. Grandma had fiery red hair and freckles she couldn't stand. She wasn't a girly girl by any means, definitely a "tomboy," but adored the one doll she owned and her frilly dresses her father brought back when he traveled to the city. Grandma loved her baby doll so much. She would sit and stare at it, not even playing with the doll. Grandma had to work very hard to earn that beloved toy. She had to get so many subscriptions to a magazine before she could send away for her adored treasure. The doll was appreciated and loved as a special family member instead of a toy. She still has it to this day, and it is in pristine condition.

Grandma Lu and her family always had plenty of food and never went without. Her mother had 13 other siblings that lived nearby, and all saw to it that the crops they farmed and the meat they raised were shared among the entire family. There was rarely a need to go to the store for food. Canning took place immediately after crops were picked and stored in a dark pantry. When it was time for dinner, Grandma's mom went to the pantry to see what foods she wanted to combine to make a meal for the evening. It was Grandma Lu's job to walk with a metal bucket to a local creamery that was all of a block away. Paying 10 cents, she would buy a glass bottle of milk, perfectly sized for fitting in her bucket.

Desserts were a special treat and were not eaten as a snack or meal. Family traditional cooking was passed from generation to generation, and generational heritage dishes were staples during the holidays. Families were an important part of life. Helping one another was a given, not a burden. Life was slower, less stressful. Life wasn't perfect, problems still existed in the world, in her family and others, but some of the significant issues with health that exist today weren't as prevalent.

Today the average family can all be living under one roof or split up due to divorce or single parenthood. Childhood memories can still be good or mixed with complications and confusions. Many toys have been put on the backburner, though the selection of toys available today is vast. Screens of all sizes have taken over and replaced the need for many toys. Screens grab our children's attention, which allows parents to get their "stuff" done without the interruptions of a child. Playing outside isn't as exciting as what screens have to offer; in some cases, outside can be a dangerous place.

Food is often grabbed at the store, not knowing where it is grown or manufactured. Meals that can be prepared quickly are a bonus, and the faster, the better. Some meals are grabbed on the go through a drive-thru, and the time we choose to eat a meal can vary according to what time is best that our schedule allows. In today's world of high tech, life is often rushed and stressful. We never seem to have enough time to get everything we need to get done. Family members are all going in different directions. Life still isn't perfect, but now, we have many health problems. We have to stop and ask ourselves, what exactly is the problem, and how can we do better?

Before we move forward, we must take a moment and think about what is going on in the world today. It's essential to look back to see how we lived in the past. In comparing the past to the present, we can see a huge difference in how we function in the world. Although we have conveniences today, some that I definitely do not care to give up, I think it's clear that some of the ways of the past may have the right answers we need to address current health problems. The nutritional content of our foods could skyrocket if we took the time to cook most of our meals at home, made with fresh local ingredients. Our relationships with our family could deepen from sitting around a table, taking time to eat meals together. Our bodies could get stronger by getting outside and walking more each day. Our health could benefit if we tweak small areas of our life and implement ideas leading back to a more basic simple time.

Take a few minutes to think about how your ancestors ate, exercised, and what their environment was like. In what ways can your family benefit from how your ancestors lived? What ideas might be good to implement in your current lifestyle to help your family become healthier?

HEALTH INFORMATION AT YOUR FINGERTIPS

"I can't wait to wake up in the morning feeling grouchy, tired, achy and out of sorts!" said NO ONE ever! None of us strive or wish to be unhealthy. Yet there is an alarming number of adults currently in the United States that are. According to the Office of Disease Prevention and Health Promotion, about half of the adult population in the US has at least one chronic disease that is related to poor diet and inactivity. These days, information about health is abundant and easily accessible. We search for a word or phrase online, and immediately something pops up on anything we want to know about how to improve ourselves and our health. Health information is available in books, podcasts, social media, videos, and many other avenues. There's only one problem! The amount of information that comes at us about what is healthy and what is not is overwhelming and can be hard to sift through.

In many cases, doctors and health experts disagree, which makes understanding health advice confusing. Many people want to be healthy but have no idea where to start with the vast amount of information. Often, it's easier to look at what everybody else is doing to decide what's best for our bodies. Hippocrates said it best "One man's food is another man's poison." The same is true for everything else in health. Health is not an exact science. It's a journey that varies from person to person. We want someone to tell us what's best, yet we overlook what we should be doing, which is listening to our body and paying attention to the clues it's giving us. We want everything in a hurry, so we follow whatever new fad or diet comes along and implement it in hopes of getting healthy. Yet in many cases, something is missing. Something inside us doesn't quite seem right. Maybe it's not working for us because we chose to listen to anyone but our bodies.

As a parent, what can you do? What health advice is best for you and your family? In the chapters ahead, we will break down what balanced health looks like and how you can individualize a plan that we can implement for your child. We will mix ideas of the past with our world today, so your family can live a happy and balanced lifestyle.

Journal Points

How did your ancestors eat, get exercise, and what was their environment like?

Which of those ways can your family benefit from implementing?

What can you do to implement those in your current lifestyle to help your family become healthier?

Final Thought

Learning from the past can be one of the best guides for the future.

SECTION 2

THE WHOLE CHILD

CHAPTER 4

NUTRITION

The first step to balanced health and behaviors starts with the nourishment of our bodies by what we eat and drink. Everything begins and ends with food and nutrition. No other category affects our bodies as food does. Every single cell in our body is affected by what we choose to put in our mouths. We are either getting stronger by our food choices or weaker, by feeding or starving our cells. Optimally, we want to nourish our cells with every drink and bite we take. How your child eats now will affect them into adulthood. It is essential as a parent to make a strong base that your child can take with them as they grow. Teaching your child starting now can help them on the journey to balanced health that will last their lifetime. It's never too late to start making healthy choices, no matter the age of yourself or your child. The perfect time is right now.

As we gear up to design a healthy program for your family, one of the most important things you can do as a parent is to help set the tone and attitude around making lifestyle changes with food. A curious attitude of wanting to explore different foods because of the benefits to the body is an awesome attitude to have. Calling a lifestyle change around food, "going on a diet," can be a set up for failure. Diets are generally thought of to help someone lose weight and are only temporary, as you have to cut or eliminate foods permanently to keep the weight off. Diets make you feel restricted, and that is never a good thing to feel and can invite rebellion. A lifestyle change encourages creativity. It makes you feel as though there are choices, and you are choosing healthy options over unhealthy ones, to live a better life. Making lifestyle choices are to enhance and help the entire family, not put a single child on a restricted diet. Your attitude as a parent must be positive and hopeful. Keep patience in your back pocket, along with persistence in the weeks ahead. Your family is worth every change that is about to come.

Food Shouldn't Be a Roller Coaster Ride

Have you hosted or attended a child's birthday party that got a little out of control? I used to get so stressed out about all my boys' birthday parties hoping everything would turn out "perfect." Birthday parties have this understood progression and order. A short activity or game is usually played after the arrival of the excited guests to get things started. Then comes some main attraction, whether it's a show, a guest, or an activity. Food is generally served after the main event, in the form of a meal or just the traditional birthday cake and ice cream, with a sugar-filled beverage to accompany it. Kids always seem to inhale a ton of birthday cake, ice cream, and juice or soda!

After the food comes, it's time for the most anticipated event for the birthday child, the opening of gifts. The guests that just consumed a bunch of sugar are expected to sit still and watch the birthday child unwrap each gift. Some kids can't contain themselves, and the next thing you know, they are running around or perhaps even opening gifts FOR the birthday child. The birthday child then has a meltdown because their friend, who is supposed to be watching them at their favorite part of the party, got too excited and started acting crazy!

I have witnessed this series of events at many children's birthday parties. Yes, I hate to say I have had this happen at some of my own children's parties. This whole situation can certainly be blamed on a sugar rush and crash. You know, where you eat a lot of sugar, run around acting crazy doing things you wouldn't normally do without consuming 70 grams of sugar all at once. Then, the next thing you know... you are exhausted and too tired to do anything. You feel grouchy, maybe even weepy, and all you really want to do is take a nap. All of this is the roller coaster effect of blood sugar.

When you hear the words Blood Sugar, do you automatically think of diabetes? You do not have to have diabetes or another medical condition to be concerned and watch blood sugar levels. Blood Sugar is simply the amount of glucose in our bloodstream at a given moment. It is important to have sustained levels, although the levels won't ever remain 100% constant. Levels will go up and down throughout the day. The amount of sugar, or glucose, is meant to slowly rise and fall with the foods that you eat and the beverages you drink. Sharp dips up and down should be avoided at all costs. These sharp dips of blood sugar can cause unpleasant symptoms in the body. If drastic changes in blood sugar continue for long periods, medical conditions such as Pre-Diabetes or even Type 2 Diabetes can surface.

When proper levels of blood sugar are not maintained in the body, the first organ to suffer is the brain. The brain relies on glucose to function correctly. Not having enough glucose essentially starves the brain. When the brain is affected, everything else in the body is then affected. Unless you have a diabetic condition and need insulin, a natural solution to sustaining level glucose can be conquered in large part, by the foods that you eat. A specific combination of food will ensure a roller coaster effect will not arise. Eating a combination of protein, fats, and carbohydrates for meals and snacks can nutritionally sustain your glucose levels.

Paying attention to the intake of sugar that goes into your body is very important. Sugar is abundant in many of the processed foods that are available to us today. Staying away from sugary laced foods or foods that turn into sugar quickly in the body can be a challenge. Eating a diet high in fresh whole foods can help keep spikes of sugar levels to a minimum.

Although foods may be the most significant influencer of blood sugar in the body, it is not the only way to affect blood sugar. Blood sugar can be affected by everything, such as how we exercise, our emotions, stress, and temperature. However, food is the greatest constant impact of blood sugar. Eating properly is so important and requires mindfulness. A small amount of planning is far better than experiencing your child having a meltdown. Monitoring blood sugar, by simply watching the foods that your child intakes, could have an enormous effect on your child's behavior. Serving meals and snacks made up of the combination of protein, fats, and carbohydrates will help your child stay in control of their own body.

Symptoms of Low Blood Sugar

Headaches	Clumsiness
Thirst	Coordination problems
Shakiness	Achy Muscles
Extreme emotions	Sweating, chills, and
Fatigue	clamminess
Intense hunger	Fast heartbeat
Feeling sick all the sudden	Nausea
A general feeling of	Color draining from skin
something not being right	Nightmare or crying during
Brain fog	sleep
Confusion	Seizure
Lack of focus	

Symptoms of High Blood Sugar

Fatigue	Weight Loss
Frequent Urination	Eyesight problems
Extreme Thirst	

THE WINNING COMBINATION

Our bodies are the vehicles we use to get around every day. They are delicate machines that require the right fuel to work correctly. Just as you wouldn't put oil in a gas tank of a car and expect it to work correctly, you can't put the wrong fuel in the body and expect it to function with proper health. Our bodies are designed to properly function with the right combination of macronutrients or proteins, carbohydrates, and fats. All meals and snacks should consist of these combinations. Proteins give the body fuel to sustain power. Fats take longer to digest and help the body sustain between meals and snacks. Carbohydrates are quicker to burn in the body, which helps to get the body moving. Different body types require different amounts of the combinations of proteins, fats, and carbohydrates. Some may need more protein and fewer carbs, or some may require more carbs and less protein. Finding the right balance is imperative to each individual.

Protein

For a child's body to grow and develop properly, adequate amounts of protein need to be eaten. Protein is the building block of growing and repairing tissue. Proteins contain amino acids, which are essential for many functions in the body. During childhood, the body needs more protein than an average adult. Just like everything else, one child may need more protein than another, due to the uniqueness of the child. If your child isn't getting enough intake of protein, it can stunt their growth. Signs of a protein deficiency may look like this in your child: hair and nails stop growing, wounds take longer to heal, bones are easily fractured, edema, weakness, anxiety, trouble sleeping, and excess appetite.

There are plenty of sources of protein that can be introduced and used in the diet. There are meat sources and plant sources. Some people do well with eating both meat and plants, some better with just plants. Finding what works best for your child is always key. A variety of sources will help your child receive the right amount of nourishment. Younger children need about 1.5 grams of protein per kilogram of weight, and older children and adults need about .8-.95 grams per kilograms.

Examples of Healthy Proteins

Artichoke	Hempseed	Red Meat
Asparagus	Kale	Rice
Beans	Lentils	Seeds
Bison	Milk	Seitan
Broccoli	Nutritional Yeast	Spelt
Brussel Sprouts	Nuts	Spinach
Cheese	Oats	Spirulina
Chia Seeds	Peas	Sweet Potatoes
Chicken	Pork	Tempeh
Eggs	Potatoes	Tofu
Fish	Quinoa	Turkey

Fats

Fats are the body's reserves of fuel or stored energy. They take longer to digest, which allows the body to have periods of sustained energy. Not all fats are created equal, though. Fats that are high in Omega 3 fatty acids are essential and are important to have in the diet. Omega 3 fatty acids can decrease inflammation, which lowers the chances of skin, autoimmune, and heart disease. They also reduce the chances of depression and anxiety. Omega 3's help increase circulation, improve nerve function, and sustain healthy blood sugar levels.

A large part of the Standard American Diet contains a type of fat called trans-fats, which are chemically altered and have no nutritional value. Trans-fats damage the body and interfere with its natural production of beneficial fatty acids. It's best to avoid low-fat versions of food and eat natural sources of healthy fats. A good variety of healthy monounsaturated, polyunsaturated, and saturated fats are best. Fats should be well balanced with what's offered on the plate, and a meal should never consist of solely fats.

Examples of Healthy Fats

Avocados	Grass-Fed Beef
Coconuts	Nuts
Eggs	Olives
Ghee	Sardines
High Quality Fish	Seeds

Carbohydrates

Carbohydrates are a quick source of energy made up of sugar and starches in food. They break down in the body as sugars to give a burst of energy, while fats and proteins are slower to act. Since the body can burn carbohydrates more efficiently, carbs should be a large part of a meal or snack.

Carbohydrates are considered essential to the body because they are the most abundant sources of our intake of vitamins, minerals, and fiber. The best type of carbs to include in the diet should come from fruits and vegetables. Fresh fruits and vegetables provide enormous benefits for the body. Besides the nutrients, these carbohydrates have the advantage of being used for medicinal properties that can help detoxify the body, boost the immune system, normalize blood sugar, ramp up energy, and help lower inflammation. Carbohydrates that are processed are the worst type to eat. Being processed, they are stripped of their nutritional qualities and will spike blood sugar levels.

A variety of colors of fruit and vegetables should be incorporated in the diet, to get a wide range of benefits. Starchy carbs such as white potatoes and corn, and fruits high in natural sugar like watermelon and grapes, should be eaten in moderation and small amounts at one time. Even though these foods are beneficial, they can spike blood sugar. On a plate, carbohydrates should take up half of the food served.

Examples of Healthy Carbohydrates

Vegetables such as:	Fruits such as:	Grains such as:	Beans and Legumes such as:
Artichoke	Apples	Amaranth	Adzuki
Asparagus	Blackberries	Brown Rice	Beans
Beets	Blueberries	Buckwheat	Black Beans
Carrots	Cantaloupe	Bulgur	Black-Eyed
Celery	Grapefruit	Corn	Peas
Cucumber	Honeydew	Millet	Butter Beans
Green Beans	Kiwi	Oats	Chickpeas
Green Leafy	Mango	Rye	Kidney
Mushrooms	Mulberries	Sorghum	Beans
Onions	Oranges	Spelt	Lentils
Potatoes	Pears	Whole Wheat	Lupins
Peppers	Pineapple	Wild Rice	Navy Beans
Squash	Raspberries		Peas
Snow Peas	Strawberries		Soybeans
Zucchini			

Water

Drinking water can help dispel fake hunger pangs, keep excess weight off and fight constipation, but it also helps improve memory, sharpen focus, and clear out brain fog. An adequate amount of water needs to be consumed to support brain function. The brain is made up of somewhere between 75%-80% water and has over 14 billion brain cells that are also made up of 75% water. As with a lack of glucose, the brain is the first organ affected by a lack of water. Dehydration of the brain restricts the blood flow and oxygen going to the brain, which affects memory, mood, concentration, and focus.

Symptoms of Dehydration of the Brain

Headaches	Short attention
Brain Fog	Confusion
Fatigue	Feeling emotional

So how much water is enough? A quick, easy way to measure how much water a person should be drinking per day is to take the weight of the individual and divide it by 2. If you weigh 130 pounds, you'll need to sip on roughly 65 oz of water throughout the day. If your child is 65 pounds, they will need about 32.5 oz of water a day.

The best time to drink water is first thing in the morning so that the water depleted through the night is replenished. The absolute best thing you can do to kick start the entire body is to drink an adequate amount of water within the first 30 minutes you are awake. The worst time to drink a lot of water is during a meal. Drinking too much weakens the stomach acid working to break up the food that is eaten. Tea, which is considered a food, is better to enjoy with a meal. Avoid having your child drink too much water before bed, which can cause frequent trips to the bathroom and sleep disruption.

ALLERGIES, SENSITIVITIES, AND INTOLERANCES

Do you ever notice how many people have adverse reactions to food these days? It's easy to go into a grocery store or restaurant and see a special section that is gluten, dairy, soy, or nut-free. I could guess that most of you know someone that must avoid a specific category of food. Their reasoning may be because of allergies, digestive upsets, hormonal issues, chronic conditions, aches, and pains, or skin conditions. In some cases, the category of food did not bother them during the first part of their life but showed up as they grew older or sicker. They may have started to investigate foods and symptoms on their own or with a medical professional.

Foods can cause us to feel energetic, and certain foods can make us feel sluggish and lethargic. Body chemistry varies from individual to individual. We can have allergies, sensitivities, or intolerances to foods and drinks. Having reactions to food happens because there is a breakdown somewhere in the body. Breakdowns can be caused by the body unable to perform typically or because the food isn't natural to the body. Today, many of our foods are manufactured with colorings, additives, and preservatives. Fruits and vegetables are sprayed with chemicals. Some of the seeds used to grow our food supply come already power-packed with a dose of chemicals. If you add those seeds to the chemicals sprayed while the plant is growing, plus the chemicals added to process or preserve the food, you now have a cocktail variety of chemicals on just one single piece of a food! The processed food we call "food", isn't even real food anymore. It's been altered and processed so much that the nutrients are stripped and taken out. Our bodies may not receive an ounce of benefit from what we think we are feeding it. Chemicals are used for several reasons. Extending shelf life, changing texture and taste, changing the coloring of our food or drinks, and to keep us craving the product are a few reasons they are used.

Some people have excellent filtering and detoxification systems in their bodies. Some people aren't so well equipped and can be what's called in toxic overloaded. Years ago, we didn't see some of the same issues we have today, because the amount of processing and chemicals in the food supply wasn't as plentiful. As chemicals build up in our detoxification system, we can become sensitive to certain foods. Our digestive system starts to breakdown. For some, a natural allergy or sensitivity is present to certain foods when we are born. Allergies are immediate and can be easy to spot. Sensitivities can be slow-growing and difficult to detect and have a whole host of symptoms. Intolerances are felt after eating a food that is upsetting to the digestive system. Sensitivities and intolerances can also be explained away without realizing that a food source is a culprit.

Allergy

An allergy to a particular food is not the same as a sensitivity or intolerance. A food allergy is an immediate response in the body to a specific category of food or ingredient. Allergies can be urgent, dangerous, and life-threatening. Anaphylactic shock can occur and can be fatal. Allergies create a response from the immune system, producing IgE antibodies, which release chemicals called histamine. Those chemicals cause an allergic reaction. Specific allergies can be diagnosed by a doctor, an Allergist, who can do a panel of skin scratch tests or a blood test. Conclusive results for allergies will result in either of these tests.

Sensitivity

A food sensitivity is a response that causes the body to react in ways it usually wouldn't towards a category of food or a specific ingredient. Sensitivities can be caused by leaky gut syndrome, chemical imbalances, and toxins, such as mold exposure or heavy metals. They are hard to catch and can wreak havoc on the body and living everyday life. Food sensitivities can take up to 3 days to develop and cause a range of symptoms from aches and pains to behavioral problems. Sensitivities can mask different conditions that look and feel like a medical disease or syndrome. Sensitivities can hide and be hard to discover. Testing can be done to figure out what the body is sensitive to. However, testing is costly, generally not covered by insurance, and not always accurate. The best test involves a food diary, an elimination diet, and adding the offender back to the diet to see if there is a true reaction.

Intolerance

An intolerance is the body's lack of ability to digest certain foods. Intolerances can be caused by a lack of enzymes, lack of hydrochloric acid, parasites, yeast, or bacteria. Intolerance testing can be done, but it is often costly and not covered by insurance companies. Ruling out allergies and sensitivities to a certain food or ingredients is best before looking into intolerances.

Leaky Gut

Children with behavioral issues can have a leaky gut. Leaky Gut Syndrome is a condition where the body is not able to digest food. Undigested particles can permeate through the intestinal lining and leak into the bloodstream and can be responsible for conditions like sensitivities and intolerances. There are many causes of Leaky Gut Syndrome, but some include unhealthy eating habits, toxins, and chronic stress. The first step in fixing a leaky gut is to eliminate any food sensitivities.

Checklist

Ruling out sensitivities is important and can make a huge difference in children's behavior. If you feel like your child may have a sensitivity reaction to food, but you are not sure what the food is, taking the following Symptoms Checklist can help.

Symptoms Checklist

Does your child have symptoms of a food sensitivity? Circle or highlight the symptoms below that you feel your child exhibits. If there are symptoms that your child has that are not on the list, write them on the lines below.

Behavior- ADD/ADHD behavior (inattentiveness, hyperactive, lack of focus, restless), OCD behaviors (obsessive and repetitive behavior), irritability, poor eye contact, food cravings, poor comprehension, anger, brain fog, aggression, lack of interest, disorganized thinking and disorientation, anxiety, depression, moodiness, over emotional, inappropriate laughter

Circulatory System- elevated blood pressure, racing heart, irregular pulse

Digestive System- upset stomach, IBS, constipation, diarrhea, mucus in stool, nausea, vomiting, gas, cramping, heartburn, bloating, abdominal pain

General- fatigue, delayed growth, delayed puberty, lethargy, speech disorders, vision problems, cravings

Neurological System- headaches, migraines, dizziness, ears ringing, tics, insomnia, night terrors, sleep disruptions

Respiratory System- coughing, sore throat, clearing throat constantly, canker sores in the mouth, bleeding or swollen gums, tooth discoloration, excess mucus, runny nose, congestion, watery or itchy eyes, sinus problems, ear infections, nasal polyps

Skeletal and Muscular System- aches and pains, swelling, stiffness

Skin- dark circles under the eyes, rosy red cheeks and ears, acne, hair loss, skin disruptions and disorders, rashes, elbow rash, eczema, hives

Urinary System- edema, bladder infections

Others:

_____

_____

_____

_____

_____

_____

_____

_____

Common Offenders That Produce Symptoms

Any Sensitivity

Aches and Pains	Heartburn
Bloating	Irregular Pulse
Coughing	Irritability
Dark Circles Under Eyes	Racing Heart
Elevated Blood Pressure	Skin Rash and Hives
Fatigue	Swelling and Stiffness
Food Cravings	Throat Clearing
	Watery Itchy Eyes

Corn

ADD/ADHD Behavior	Lack of Concentration
Aggression	Lack of Focus
Anger	Moodiness
Anxiety	Night Terrors
Behavior Problems	OCD Behavior
Brain Fog	Skin Disruption and
Headaches	Disorders
Hyperactivity	Sleep Disruptions
	Tics

Dairy/Soy/Casein

Acne	Frequent Sinus Infections
Anxiety	IBS Constipation/Diarrhea
Behavioral Issues	Inappropriate Laughter
Brain Fog	Lack of Interest
Congestion	Mucus in Stools
Depression	Poor Comprehension
Eczema	Poor Eye Contact
Excess Mucus	Repetitive Behavior
Frequent Ear	Rosy Red Cheeks or Ears
Infections	Runny Nose
	Sore Throat

Gluten

ADD/ADHD	Eczema
Behavior	Elbow Rash
Anxiety	Frequent Bladder Infections
Bleeding or Swollen	Headaches
Gums	Inappropriate Laughter
Brain Fog	Lack of Interest
Canker Sores	Nausea
Constipation	Over Emotional/Moodiness
Cramping	Poor Comprehension
Delayed Growth	Poor Eye Contact
Delayed Puberty	Repetitive Behavior
Diarrhea	Tooth Discoloration
	Vomiting

Additives- Preservatives/Dyes/Flavor Enhancers/Fragrances

Abdominal Pain	Hyperactivity
Acne	Insomnia
Aggression	Lack of Concentration
Behavior Problems	Lack of Focus
Congestion	Lethargy
Disorganized Thinking	Migraines
Disorientation	Mood Swings
Dizziness	Nasal Polyps
Ear Infection	Nausea
Eczema	Ringing in Ears
Edema	Skin Rash
Gas	Speech Disorder
Headaches	Tics
Heartburn	Upset Stomach
Hives	Vision Problems

(Please note, symptoms can vary in each individual.)

QUALITY OF FOOD

Organic, local, and Non-GMO are excellent choices of types of food to buy and serve your family. If you are not buying foods and beverages in these categories, chances are your food is filled with additives such as preservatives and chemicals. People can eat foods and not feel an immediate reaction from the additives, but somewhere down the road, the effects can surface. Feeding your children foods with additives can ultimately set them up for toxic overload.

Organic

Organic foods are foods that are grown without the use of antibiotics, hormones, or pesticides. Some foods should be bought only organic, while others are considered to be safe to eat non-organic. Two lists that are helpful to follow are called the "The Dirty Dozen" and "The Clean Fifteen." These are great guides to help you decide what foods should be bought organically and what non-organic foods are safe to purchase. However, buying fruits and vegetables that are not organic doesn't ensure the freshness, nutrient content, or that they hold absolutely no chemicals.

Having the word organic on the label does tend to make the item cost more. With a little planning and creativity, these foods can be cost-effective for a budget. If you are a struggling parent that is challenged by stretching your money for meals, know that a good variety of choices are out there for you. I struggled for a time, and I definitely had to stretch meals for my family of five as far as they could go, without compromising or giving into foods that were not safe. Home-cooked meals, although they do cost your time, will end up saving you big money in the end. Cooking in large batches, freezing ingredients, and utilizing leftovers can help extend your budget.

Local

Buying local is a great way to save money and eat freshly. Farmer's Markets provide fresh local homegrown foods and often other products such as lotions, essential oils, candles, and flowers. Co-ops are available in many communities. Buying into a co-op can ultimately save big bucks, but foods are picked and divided according to what is grown and in season. Buying seasonally fresh local food is an amazing way to eat, and I highly encourage it! A co-op is something to consider, especially if you are on a limited budget. Be sure to investigate Farmer's Markets and Co-op's available in your area to decide what works best for your family.

GMO

GMO stands for a genetically modified organism. GMOs have only been in our food supply for the last 20 years. Some countries have banned GMOs because too little is known about the effects. GMOs have been shown in studies to create allergic responses, damage intestinal walls in the body, and impair digestion. Foods that are Non-GMO come with labels and are the safest choice.

Dirty or Clean?

The Dirty Dozen

Strawberries

Spinach

Nectarines

Apples

Peaches

Pears

Cherries

Grapes

Celery

Tomatoes

Sweet Bell Peppers

Potatoes

The Clean Fifteen

Sweet Corn

Avocado

Pineapple

Cabbage

Onions

Sweet Peas

Papaya

Asparagus

Mango

Eggplant

Honeydew

Kiwi

Cantaloupe

Cauliflower

Broccoli

Journal Points

What would you like to improve about your child's diet?

Final Thought

"Healing is a matter of time, but it is sometimes also a matter of opportunity."

-Hippocrates

CHAPTER 5

PHYSICAL FITNESS

Just as we eat food for nourishment, we must nourish our body with exercise to stay physically fit. You can bet if your child isn't getting the right amount of exercise their body needs, they will not be at their best every day. Not getting enough exercise could even cause your child to have behavioral problems. Some benefits of keeping your child physically fit include releasing pent up energy, stimulation of the brain, and keeping the body strong. Forming regular exercise habits now with your child will ensure healthy behavior and an active, healthy lifestyle for them, later in life.

CHANGE THE MIND

If you ask your kids if they want to exercise, chances are the answer will be no. Exercise can have a negative connotation attached to it. When I was a child, I thought exercise meant going to P.E. class, which I dreaded participating in. During my freshman and sophomore year of high school, one unit in P.E. was swimming. I really dreaded that! I was a good swimmer, and I enjoyed the activity. However, I did not enjoy being seen in a swimsuit in front of my class. I felt completely AWKWARD! I was too focused on what others would think of my body instead of focusing on having fun and enjoying the benefits of what swimming could offer my body. This whole swimming scenario pretty much sums up how I used to view exercise. I may have enjoyed some of the activities, but at the same time, I felt awkward because of how my body looked and that I wouldn't be good enough at the activity to participate. These ideas I had in my mind shaped my view of exercise that I brought into adulthood.

For many years I did not exercise. It wasn't until I felt a decline in my health before I started some form of regular fitness. I started with basic activities like walking. Walking led me to run, which led me to swim, bike, weight train, and even try frisbee golf. I also learned how to do Yoga, Pilates, and started hiking. Now, I could make a long list of activities I would love to try! So, what changed? My views about exercise. I learned that being physically fit not only helped my body stay strong, but also gave me more energy. My mind became more alert, and I felt great! Your child may have a similar view of exercise, as I did when I was young. Exercise is so much more than an emotion of feeling awkward about participation, what your body currently looks like, and not being good enough. With a few shortcuts, you can help your child change their view about what physical fitness means, just like I did.

To Each His Own

If I asked my 15 year old son Benji if he would like to join me in a mile walk around the block with mountain views and fresh air, I can assure you the answer would be no. I can see it now; his whole demeanor would change right after he heard two words "mile walk." His shoulders would slump, he'd hang his head, and with a long face, he would say to me, "I don't really want to." However, if I asked him if he would like to go practice marching while playing his trumpet on a summer day in the 100-degree heat of the Arizona desert, his answer would be, "let me get my trumpet!" I can tell you for sure, I'd much rather walk a mile than march with a trumpet any day, but our ideas of fun and exercise differ.

Physical Fitness is individual. What may be fun for you may not be fun for your child! There are so many ways to become fit and maintain health. The goal is to get your child active and involved with a form of exercise they enjoy. Nothing is concrete. Your child doesn't have to perform a task in a certain way for an activity to be called exercise. In fact, trying a wide variety of exercises can help your child pick and choose what they would like to do. Exercise does not have to mean doing activities that you dread, and it doesn't have to be mundane or boring. Exercise SHOULD be something we all look forward to as fun, a challenge, and a stress release. It should never be a chore or looked at as punishment.

Fun Ideas of Exercise

Homemade obstacle course- Build an obstacle course with items around the house or have your child build an obstacle course. Pillows can become leap pads, strings become beams to walk on, guns that shoot foam bullets can be used with a homemade shooting range, the opportunities are endless!

Not your traditional game of tag- Sometimes, when my second son would walk home from his middle school bus stop, I would find a place to hide. I would wait excitedly for him, either inside or outside the house. Eventually, he would walk by, and I would jump out and yell, "YOU'RE IT!" and tag him. We would run around until he caught me, and that concluded the short game of tag. No way could I ever tag that kid back; he was way too quick. I HAD to hide to catch him. It became a great way to enjoy a short burst of exercise that got us both sprinting and a fun way to bond.

Scavenger Hunt- This was one of my favorite games to play with the kids when they were younger! It also makes a great indoor game for rainy days. I would make each child a list of items around the house like rubber bands, an acorn, a picture of a rainbow, a ruler, a yellow crayon, and so on. Whoever found everything on their list first, won the game. The kids would run around the house trying to find everything, burning energy without even realizing it!

Benefits to the body

If you tell your child to run down the street and back because it is healthy, they may not be inclined to do what you ask. If you ask them to run down the street and back, but instead say running will help you grow taller, they may feel more motivated to do the exercise. Helping your child to understand that being physically fit will help their body function better, can change their outlook on exercise. Instead of saying "exercise because it's good for you" or "you need to exercise, so you don't gain weight," tell them a fact like growing children need impact on bones to help them grow taller. Share with your child the chart in this Chapter showing what exercise can do for the different areas of the body.

Bones, Joints and Muscles-

The body was designed to move. We have joints, hinges, and muscles that need to be exercised every single day. Bones grow from impact, joints strengthen to hold up under stress, and muscles lengthen and strengthen. Children need more exercise than adults to help stimulate their growing bones. Circulation is improved when exercising, which is vital to a muscle we can't live without, the heart. With improved circulation, oxygen levels in the body will increase, which helps the lungs stay strong.

Digestion-

Exercise can significantly help with gastrointestinal issues such as low stomach acid, constipation, gas, and any digestion process stuck on slow. Working the core part of the body can release pent up gas bubbles and help move along digestion and bowel movements.

Immune System-

Regular exercise can help your child stay healthy and keep from catching illnesses. The immune system improves with activity by supporting the body to stay healthy and strong naturally. The lymphatic system is like a garbage collector. The last thing you want to happen is for the lymph nodes to get clogged. Exercise releases the lymph to help keep everything moving and flowing as it should be. Jumping on a trampoline is an excellent way to release any toxic build-ups (and a great way to release cellulite).

Skin-

An adequate amount of exercise also can help with acne. Sweating is the best way to detoxify the body's largest organ, the skin. Exercise helps to balance out blood sugar, open pores, and relieve stress, which can all be causes of acne.

Brain-

Exercise isn't just beneficial for the mechanical uses of the body. Exercise promotes circulation throughout our

body and stimulates the brain. If your child ever has a homework crisis leaving them feeling frustrated and stuck, a good dose of exercise can do wonders. We do some of our best thinking while exercising! Creativity and focus abound through us with activity. Simply taking a walk outside can create a whole other dynamic for our moods, thoughts, and memory.

Moods and Behavior-

Feeling healthy about our bodies is important to people of all ages. During the sensitive time of the pre-teen and teenage years, exercise can help with self-esteem and moodiness. Feel-good chemicals or endorphins are released with physical activity. Moods balance out, anxiety is lowered, and depression can become curtailed.

Exercise and the Body

Helps the brain to think clearer
and be creative

Reduces acne breakouts

Strengthens the heart and
lungs

Promotes digestion

Helps us from getting
sick

Stimulates bones

HOW MUCH IS ENOUGH

To maintain balanced health, a suggested length of exercise time is an hour a day, according to the U.S. Department of Health and Human Services. Sixty minutes a day can ensure your child is getting enough activity. The length of exercise time can be continuous or divided throughout the day. Doing short exercise movements in segments can all add up at the end of the day.

Varying types of activities is GOOD for the body, heart, and soul. An assortment of exercises will give your child an opportunity for a range of experiences and to see what kind of movement they enjoy. The list of possibilities is never-ending! Exercises can be done in a group or alone. They can be done inside or outside in a variety of ways. Look at physical fitness as a chance for creativity. Playing a game of tag can be counted as an exercise, but the child is just having fun! Exercise needs to be viewed as a chance to have fun, build the body, and maybe even have a little friendly competition and bonding time. Positive experiences with exercise and seeing the benefits will ensure the child continues into adulthood with physical fitness.

Journaling Points

What are some ways you can incorporate exercise into your everyday routine with your family?

What new types of activities can you introduce?

Final Thought

"To keep the body in good health is a duty... otherwise we shall not be able to keep our mind strong and clear."

-Gautama Buddha

CHAPTER 6

SLEEP AND MEDITATION

There was a short time in my life, where I was only getting 4-5 hours of sleep each night. During that time, my health was suffering, and I didn't feel good most of the time. I was always tired, and my blood sugar was constantly up and down. I wasn't feeling as bubbly and happy as I once felt. Getting out of bed in the morning was extremely hard during that time, which was unusual because I am a morning person. I got to the point where I was tired of being tired. I made a commitment to myself to conquer this area of my life and get more sleep. After a few short days of a good night's sleep, I started to feel so much better. My mood improved, I had more energy, and my blood sugar did not fluctuate as much. I couldn't believe what an extra 2 hours of sleep a night did for my health. It's one of those times where you know you should get more sleep, but you don't necessarily buy into that your health could drastically improve if you only went to bed earlier. I was newly divorced and had a lot going on in my life. Being a busy mom, I sacrificed my sleep for things like housework, checking emails, doing paperwork, and my downtime. I also sacrificed sleep for worrying about my children, the future, bills, and even how to improve my health. I have felt firsthand how sleep deprivation can drastically affect your health, and I have benefitted from feeling how the right amount of sleep can improve health in a big way. If your child lacks sleep, this could be a gamechanger on the health, behavior, and moods of your child.

SLEEP AND THE BODY

Not only does lack of sleep give your child a serious case of the grumpies, but it also causes their body to underperform. There are direct connections between health and sleep. During sleep, critical activities take place like rest, recovery, and repairing of the body. With continuous proper sleep, we can expect to have an increase in energy levels, make better choices, improved concentration, focus and moods, and reduced anxiety. During sleep, a critical function of the brain takes place called memory consolidation. Memory consolidation allows the brain to store and learn at an optimum level. Hormones are also regulated, and the growth of muscles takes place during sleep. By the morning, your child's body is ready for the new day. So many essential processes happen during the sleep cycle; it is vital to protect and preserve sleep.

Children crave and need routine in all areas of their life. It helps them to feel safe, provided for, and to understand what is expected of them. Children need the routine of a sleep schedule for their bodies. The body is on a natural rhythm of its own, and it needs to be guided and followed. The human body has a natural sleep and wake cycle called the circadian rhythm. When it is dark outside, naturally, it is time for the body to start preparing for sleep. During daylight, it is naturally time to be awake. Staying on this cycle makes it easier to get good quality sleep. This is because sunlight stimulates a hormone called melatonin, which our body needs to produce in order to sleep.

To promote the body's natural rhythms, as a parent, you can do a few things to help. The first thing you can do is make sure during the daytime that your child gets enough movement and exercise. Limiting caffeine throughout the day and eliminating it in the late afternoon and evening can ensure the body is free from the stimulate to keep your child awake. Next, stick to a schedule or routine at night, limit screen exposure in the evening, and help your child do calming activities before bed. Bedtime should be a time to enjoy your child and not a screaming stressful way to end the night.

There are specific things that negatively affect the natural rhythm. Some of these include not getting enough sun exposure, getting too much extra light at night, exercising or eating late at night, and drinking too much before bed. The most important thing parents can do is to keep a regular sleep schedule and routine for their child. If you do not have one, or it is continuously changing, it is time to think of sleep as necessary as eating and drinking.

How much sleep is necessary?

Newborns 14-18 hours	School Age Children
Infants 12-15 hours	9-11 hours
Toddlers 11-14 hours	Teens 8-10 hours
Preschoolers 10-13 hours	Adults 7-9 hours
	Older Adults 7-8 hours

Sleep and the Body

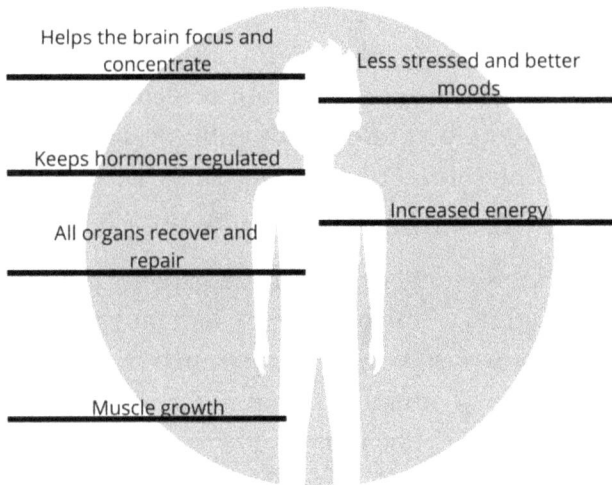

Helps the brain focus and concentrate

Less stressed and better moods

Keeps hormones regulated

Increased energy

All organs recover and repair

Muscle growth

MEDITATION

I can imagine some of you that are reading this book, came upon this section of meditation, and perhaps a few sarcastic thoughts have come to your mind about not being able to get your child to meditate. Back when Braeden was having behavioral problems, I'm pretty sure if somebody would've told me to have him meditate, I would have thought that person was out of their mind! I could never imagine Braeden sitting still, crossing his legs, closing his eyes, and being quiet for any amount of time other than when he was sleeping. I would have thought meditation was a joke, and I was the one that needed the quiet meditation time, not him! What I didn't understand back then was that meditation soothes and feeds the brain. Meditation also helps control the body and the mind. Meditation could have helped Braeden feel in control when his body was going out of control. It would have given him a tool to fall back on, a "go-to" when he felt angry and didn't know why or how to express it. Children ultimately want to please their parents, and they do not like the overwhelming feeling of anger or the waves of sadness and guilt. Meditation is an amazing tool that, in conjunction with the other tools in this book, is not to be underestimated.

Meditation has a stereotype to be weird or only for super health nuts or spiritual people. Everyone should learn how and why we need to meditate daily to help our brain and our entire body. Learning this skill as a child will give them an advantage. At an elementary school in Baltimore, instead of giving children detention when they got in trouble, they did something radically different. Educators decided to show the children how to do a meditation in what they call a Mindful Moment Room. Students sent to the room talked about why they were there, then did breathing exercises. The results were astonishing. Children learned when they felt themselves get out of control, they could stop, take a short break, breathe, and start over. Because they learned how to deal with any stress they felt, the program led to the results of fewer children receiving disciplinary actions, and even the school attendance increased.

As the school in Baltimore has demonstrated, relaxing the mind has many benefits. It calms the mind and redirects it to be able to focus and concentrate. Rhythmic breathing exercises relax the sympathetic nervous system, which is our fight or flight response. The exercises help lower cortisol levels in the body, our stress hormones. One study shows that meditation dramatically reduces anxiety symptoms and is a promising intervention for attention and behavior problems.

We all need time alone to recharge and relax. Without meditation, we can get anxious, feel detached, and have an overall feeling of being overwhelmed. The goal of meditation is to be able to find a way for your child to release any pent-up emotions or energy. They will then be able to think clearer and calm themselves, which will naturally lead to better behavior. When we are running on empty, often in the middle of the day, meditation can be the perfect way to recharge and begin the second half of the day. It's that short timeout that can make a world of difference.

Meditation is practiced in many ways and can be individualized to fit the needs of each child. It can be done through gentle exercises such as stretching or yoga, reading a book, guided meditation, visual imagery, or breathing exercises. Teaching and practicing a calming technique can make a massive impact on your child as an adult. It can give them a go-to stress release in an all too demanding world.

Journal Points

Does your child have a bedtime routine? If so, what is it?

What type of meditation would work best for your child?

Final Thought

"The best cure for the body is a quiet mind."

-Napoleon Bonaparte

CHAPTER 7

THE MIND

WE ARE WHAT WE THINK

We all have that little voice in our head that interjects thoughts at the most inconvenient times. The tone of the voice is generally never pleasant and can say things such as, "That was dumb," "No one likes you," "Why can't you do things right." It can come up with endless lies, rather quickly too! It's so important to shut that voice off, the earlier in your child's life, the better. The voice needs to be taught how to be your child's best friend instead of an enemy. Equipping your child with this can radically change how your child views themselves.

There is a small part in the back of our brains called the amygdala. As a child, the amygdala makes up rules, or truths, that we live by as we grow. The "truths" don't have to be *truthful,* but they are true to that person. As an example, if a young child was scared by a dog, that child may continue to fear all dogs because the amygdala held the fear of the incident with one dog. Another example is of a young girl who was shamed by a trusted member of her family. She was told that she was fat and shouldn't wear shorts. Hearing this, led her to believe she was not the weight she should be. The amygdala will hold onto that "truth" until it is replaced with a new truth. So, that little girl went on for years believing and seeing herself as fat, when really, she was average size and not overweight.

In both examples, the children are holding onto an old pattern of a learned thought, affecting outlooks and behaviors. The fantastic news is the old thoughts simply must be replaced with a new truth! In a loving, healthy environment, the amygdala can update itself. It can also be updated with a few exercises. For the girl that believes she is overweight, first, it must be identified; she thinks she is overweight. Next, she can replace that thought with something else, such as I am healthy, strong, and beautiful. Now the brain has something positive to work with! Whatever you present to the mind, it will try to figure out how to become or do the thought. If you say to yourself, I am fat, and the brain will say, yes, I am fat and support bad habits that can take place to become overweight. "I can't exercise. I am too fat. I can't wear shorts. I am too fat. I don't make friends easily, because I am too fat." Guilt, sadness, loneliness, anxiety, and depression can take over, even at a young age. Negative thoughts create negative self-esteem and outlooks on life. Positive thoughts create healthy self-esteem and a great outlook on life.

Many thoughts run through our heads all day long like a broken recording. Have you ever asked your child what they think about? Our children must meditate on positive, helpful thoughts instead of negative, self-defeating ones our inner voice may tell us. Negative thoughts scientifically have been shown to change the chemistry in the brain. With happy thoughts, endorphins release in the brain. Endorphins are hormones that make us feel happy. When we think positive, we feel good. When we think a thought that is angry or sad, we become angry or sad. Negative thoughts can be picked up as baggage. Pretty soon, we can become overloaded with a bunch of baggage, without remembering where it all came from. The quicker we let go of the baggage, the easier it is to move through life.

Mistakes are Golden

All of us have been in uncomfortable situations when we have made a mistake that left us feeling ashamed, embarrassed, sad, and guilty. After a mistake happens, we wonder why we couldn't have done better or why we didn't do anything differently. I'm here to let you know, mistakes never need to hold our children or us prisoner to negative feelings again. Mistakes are like gold. Of course, I am not suggesting making mistakes on purpose, but accidents and mistakes are learning curves. We learn some of the best lessons from the mistakes we've made!

Children explore the world and learn boundaries by making mistakes. Some kids are good listeners and heed the advice of their parents, and a good amount of kids are "ME DO" kids. What's that you ask? A "Me Do" kid is one of those children that no matter what you tell them, they will do things their way. I had a child like this, my second son Jensen. If I told him not to touch something because it was hot, sure enough, he'd be right there touching it and burning his finger. He was the King of the Me Do's when he was little. I could always count on Jensen to do the exact opposite of what I asked him to do, especially if it was dangerous. Danger seemed to challenge and ignite this kid!

After many learning experiences, Mr. Me Do started to understand that listening to his mom might save him from some hurtful lessons. Now, Mr. Me Do did make appearances during Jensen's teenage years, and once again, lessons from mistakes were learned on his own. That's just the point, learning. Mistakes are meant to be learned from. If a child isn't making mistakes, or an adult for that matter, we should start wondering if they are participating in life! Mistakes can humble us, make us sensitive to other's feelings, and connect us to the world and living things in it. They can save us from losing money in the future, keep us from procrastination, help us love people, teach us forgiveness, and so much more. Mistakes need to be explained as this and not as a chance to shame or be harsh on our children.

Journal Points

Ask your child what thoughts play over and over in their head.

Ask your child how they view themselves.

Did any of the answers surprise you?

Final Thought

"The mind is everything. What you think you become."

-Gautama Buddha

CHAPTER 8

THE ENVIRONMENT

WHAT SURROUNDS US

Our environment is everything that surrounds us, including the people, places and all other things. When we talk about the environment and our health, there are so many aspects involved. In this book, I have included a few significant factors of the environment that can make a huge difference and impact on our children, their behavior, and how they grow.

RELATIONSHIPS

Not all of us are born into an ideal family that has two loving parents that are happy to be together. Not all of us have families that grow together to be strong, healthy, and bonded in a relationship. I know I didn't grow up that way, even though my parents were married until I was 20 years old. Unfortunately, neither did my children. Their father and I divorced when my boys were 14, 11, and 7. I didn't know what a healthy partner relationship looked like until after I got divorced. Not the ideal time to show my children the definition of a strong, healthy relationship. However, I couldn't give them something I didn't know how to do back then.

In my singlehood, I did learn and help them to see what a healthy relationship looks like. The point is, we all lack, and no one is perfect. Your child isn't trying to get perfection from you. Your child wants what we all look for in a relationship. Children want to know that they are free to be themselves and will be loved no matter what. They want to be needed, helped, and guided. They want to be free to express themselves, to trust that you to have their best interests at heart, and know that no matter what, you are there for them. You may not always love their behavior, but you love them for being the person they were born to be. Your children want to know that you believe and see the best in them and not just their failures.

So, Mom and Dad, Caregiver, if this is who you are or who you are striving to be for your child, you are doing amazingly awesome. You don't have to be perfect; you won't be perfect. You are ok, and you are on your way to becoming better, just as your children are. You are the most important person that will model a relationship for them, so be the best you! Your children will grow up seeing what a healthy, loving relationship should look like in a parent, in a friendship, and in partnership.

SCREENS

When I was taking a History class in college, I had to write a paper on World War II. I decided to interview my Grandpa and his identical twin, who enlisted in the Navy during the War. I learned fascinating information about them and saw interactions between them that were priceless. I heard stories about being so connected as twins; they were able to feel one another's pain. I heard about them both contracting illnesses, even though they were on different ships and in different parts of the world at the same time. All their war stories painted pictures in my head, but not like a picture I could get from reading a book. I was able to hear the fluctuations in their voices and the emotions behind the stories. I could hear and see the good memories, like the time the two of them went AWOL to visit one another because they heard both were at the same port at the same time. (They received a night in the brig for the offense, but they said it was well worth it.) I also saw the heavyweight and burden of the bad, when they looked away in the distance with a long stare, avoiding questions of fighting in World War II.

The interactions between the two were indescribable during the interview. I totally could see how they fed off of each other. It was like they were a comedy team and I was the audience or maybe the victim, I'm not quite sure. Had I been in college today writing a paper about World War II, I would have simply done the research online and written the paper. I wouldn't have taken the time to find and interview someone from the War. It's easier to read about someone's experience. Had I done that; I would have missed one of the fondest memories I have of my Grandpa today.

Screens have taken over personal connections and interactions and have entertained us right out of valuable personal experiences. They have made life easier and less complex. They have given us instant gratification; we can have anything at our fingertips.

Screens have given us great distractions. We can learn more and quicker, with information that comes at us in a flash. Screens have also shown our children information and images that we wouldn't want them to see. Screens have taught us to have a short attention span and how to be impatient. Screens have also taught us how to ignore people and situations. At some point, enough is enough, and a balance needs to be struck with boundaries.

Screens are not horrible, but how we use them can be. As adults, we need to model for our children what is a good use of our time and what is a drain. Absolutely technology is incredible, but we need to use it in the right way. Sitting on a screen texting, playing, or catching up on social media as your child sits with you, can have opposite effects that you may not realize. In no way am I suggesting not to use your phone around your children. I am saying we need to be mindful of how much we use our phones in front of our children. If your teen walks in a room and you are on your phone doing "important things," it's time to put it down and have a conversation with them. Even though they may only have two words to say to you, just being present with them can be monumental. Connecting with your children is so important and needs to be developed over time. All the little interactions do add up. So, put down the screen and encourage your child to do the same.

CHEMICALS

Having sensitivities is not just limited to the food we eat, but we can have sensitivities to the everyday environment around us. Chemicals are likely in our homes, schools, and everywhere we go. Chemicals can be in cleaning products, sprays, candles, yard treatment, air fresheners, perfumes, laundry products, sheets, clothing, toys, cars, water, and pools. It is tough to escape the use of chemicals in our environment. We cannot control every setting we are in; however, we can reduce our exposure in our homes. Reducing our exposure to chemicals will help lessen the burden of toxic overload on the body.

Chemicals can stimulate physical symptoms along with behavioral problems. Braeden experiences tics with exposure to chemicals. Tics or habits, as we called them, are involuntary movements that can involve any part of the body, including sounds or verbal mimicking. Braeden's tics have varied, but some of the tics are stretching his arms out, clearing his voice, a faint whistle, and the blinking of his eyes. If you have had a child with tics, you understand how hard and sometimes even painful it can be to watch.

Chemicals in the air are one trigger of Braeden's tics. Some of those chemicals come from walking in buildings that have an overpowering cleaning product smell or schools heavily deodorized with sprays. Braeden and Benji went to an elementary school like this. The school had open concept rooms that were not individually divided with walls. Instead, classes had dividers to section the rooms from one another throughout most of the school. Teachers were free to burn candles, spray air freshener, and use plug-in scented deodorizers. Yes, it helped freshen the air, which can be done without the use of chemicals, but it also triggered Braeden to have tics. We can't control other people and their choices to use products with damaging chemicals, but we can control what we put into our immediate environment. Limiting the use of chemicals and the environments that have them, will lessen the toxic overload on your child.

Symptoms of chemical exposures can cause fatigue, muscle aches and pains, headaches, rashes, brain fog, lack of focus, tics and tremors, sneezing, watery eyes, chest pain, asthma, and hyperactivity.

TOXINS

Toxin exposure differs from chemical exposure, although the symptoms can be the same. They can come from inside the body from waste that is created by bacteria, fungus, or parasites. They can also come from outside the body, float in the air, be ingested, or inhaled. Toxins create chaos within the body and can be hard to diagnose and get rid of, especially if you do not know what you are fighting. Prolonged exposure to toxins can bring on conditions that affect the brain, muscles, immune system, and set off allergic reactions. Nutrition, exercise, and good quality of sleep play a role in how the body deals with toxins. Cleaning up those areas will produce positive effects on the body; however, if you are continually exposed to a specific toxin, it will need to be addressed to make a full recovery.

Black Mold

Black mold is dangerous and can be downright debilitating. Mold exposure is more common than you may realize. It can be daunting, especially on a day to day basis without realizing the exposure. Mold needs to be eradicated to heal from it. Regularly inspect your home for any water leaks or damage. Showers, toilets, and sinks should be free from mold. Black mold is not only damaging to homes but is very damaging to people.

Mold exposure symptoms can include fatigue, brain fog, achy muscles, chronic infections, congestion, asthma-like symptoms, arthritis-like symptoms, night sweats, tics, and tremors.

Candida

Does your child have a history of thrush, athlete's foot, yeast infections, or antibiotic use? They could very well have an overgrowth of yeast in their body. Yeast is another toxin that can create havoc. It is a webbing that grows and thrives in and on the human body. It can grow anywhere. Yeast drills through tissue and can leave holes in our intestines creating Leaky Gut Syndrome. Yeast can become resistant to treatments and be hard to eradicate. When treating yeast, different natural products must be used diligently and alternated to create resistance from taking place. An overgrowth of yeast can be easier to spot on the body than some of the other toxins. However, discovering it inside the body is not as easy.

An overgrowth of yeast can look like yellowing of nails, peeling skin, cradle cap on the head, areas of itchiness, redness, dandruff, rashes, yeast-like discharge, sugar cravings, leaky gut syndrome, fatigue, low thyroid, allergies, and sensitivities.

Heavy Metals

Heavy metal exposure can be from the silver fillings placed in the teeth, our drinking water, in our soils where food grows, eating fish, paints, preservatives, cleaning products, bakeware, and more. If the body is holding on to any heavy metals, it can be challenging to get rid of yeast, parasites, and bacteria. Chelation is a process that helps to remove heavy metals in the body. Removal can be done naturally with foods that bind with the heavy metals.

Heavy metal exposure causes symptoms of sensitivities, allergies, brain fog, loss of concentration, confusion, chronic infections, hyperactivity, forgetfulness, and attention problems.

CLUTTER

Have you ever walked into a messy room, where there was so much to organize you didn't know where or how to start? It's like being so overwhelmed that your brain shuts off. You end up doing nothing or very little because it's easier to procrastinate and forget about it than it is to step up and start cleaning. Similarly, this is how children feel with too much clutter or selection in their environment. If your child's room or playroom is unorganized, they may not know what to play with. They may disregard most of the toys and only play with one or two things on a consistent basis. Stuffed rooms may not even have enough room for a child to play in! Telling them they must clean up the room, may overwhelm them because if it is disorganized, they may not know where anything goes. Having too many toys can be overwhelming, resulting in your child, not playing with anything.

Playing is essential to the child. It helps them learn and practice, play out scenarios, and play different roles. Building, creating, and designing is the way children learn how to be adults. It's good for their brains and their body. It helps them figure out skills they are good at and what they enjoy. It's important to keep our belongings organized, so children don't get overwhelmed. What places in your home need organization? If your first answer to that question is the whole house, it's ok! We will get there.

Journal Points

What types of chemicals do you currently use in your home?

What products would you like to find a safer alternative to use?

Does your child show any symptoms of toxins like mold, candida, or heavy metals?

What places in your house need organization?

Final Thought

A child will become a reflection of their environment.

SECTION 3

PARENTING THE WHOLE CHILD PROGRAM

CHAPTER 9

PROGRAM OVERVIEW

WHERE TO BEGIN

After breaking down the specific categories of health, it's easier to understand that we thrive when we have our needs met. Meeting a child's fundamental needs makes it easier for that child to behave better because they feel healthier. You may be thinking, sure, all this sounds great, but it's easier to read than to get my child to do any of this! I completely understand and it is OK! Looking at the whole picture of change can be very overwhelming. Any transformation can be uncomfortable, but the trick to making it go smoothly is taking small steps. Small steps not only take the stress off parenting but allows for an actual lifestyle change to take place that will sustain for a lifetime. Taking on too much at one time can be defeating and only have short term effects. In Section 3 of the book, we will take the small steps needed to make a healthy lifestyle unique to your family. Stick with the process, and you will have a happier child and a happier home. Let's get started with some guidelines to follow!

Guideline #1 Stick to the Plan

There is an order of progression to follow during this transformative program. When going through the process, it is best to stick with the order that is laid out. When you are reading the Chapters ahead, follow the directions of the Steps. The Steps will take you on a journey that includes observing, acting, and adjusting to a healthy lifestyle. All take time, commitment, and follow-through.

Think about this process as if you were building a house. First, a drawing of a plan or a blueprint is drafted. The plan or blueprint of a home can be designed to fit the needs of the family, according to rules and guidelines. As you start the building of the house, you may find a few things that need to be adjusted, but for the most part, you stick to the plan as closely as possible.

Next, laying a solid foundation, firm enough to hold the weight of a house, is vital. Without this strong foundation, the walls of the house could crumble or become weak and ultimately wouldn't hold the house in the long run. Then comes the building of the frame of the house. The frame holds the doors, windows, walls, and the roof firmly in place. Although the house looks complete on the outside, work still needs to be done inside, like painting and decorating. As you live in the house, you may want to redo a few things like repainting or landscaping the yard. With all these stages of progress, it's understandable, they go in a specific order, or it just doesn't make sense. You can't paint the walls of the house if they aren't built yet. You can't build walls without a solid foundation.

Much in the way of building a house, this is how we structure the work to be done on building a better family lifestyle. A blueprint will be made to fit the needs of your family. We will create a foundation by observing foods that are eaten and how they benefit or negatively affect your child. Then we can begin to add more foods that improve health and behavior. Next, we will check our blueprint and see the progress we made after laying the foundation. If we are on task, we can finish building the house by adding the walls and roof. The walls and roof of a healthy lifestyle are made of physical fitness, quality sleep and meditation, the mind, and the environment. As we go along, we may have to make adjustments with varieties of food or the types of exercises we do, but because we laid a strong foundation, didn't rush or skip steps, we know our house can withstand the changes and come out beautifully.

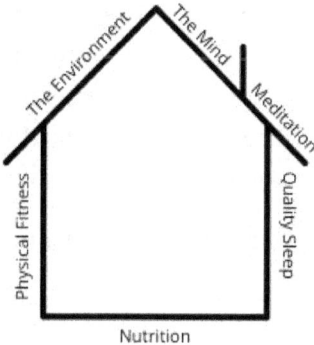

Guideline #2 Be the Change

Children learn best by example. Your child waits, wants, and depends on you to guide them in life. This process isn't something they can do on their own. The best way to change the whole family's lifestyle is to have everyone participate. Don't single out your child or ever treat this program as a form of punishment for your child's bad behavior. Be the change you want to see in your child! Start with you, and you'll be surprised at the trickle-down effect it will have on your family. I will be here as your guide for information and support, so you may guide and teach your children how to improve their behavior and health while feeling amazing doing it.

Guideline #3 Commit

To ensure success with the program, make a commitment to yourself and your child that you will follow through with this journey. I know how difficult parenting a child with bad behavior consistently can be. However, it is more challenging to go through life trying to fix behaviors than it is to try to meet a child's basic needs. Do not give up on yourself and never give up on your child. You were given your child for a reason, stay strong, and carry on. You can do this!

Guideline #4 The Do's and Don'ts of the Program

Do:

Stick with changing one area of health at a time. Do not try to tackle everything at once. That is way too overwhelming, and it can set you up for a fail. Slow and steady, stay the course. Small steps may seem insignificant, but they are the key to transforming lifestyles.

Celebrate all the small successes! Take time to cheer yourself and your child on with every little positive change.

Educate yourself. Start reading about subjects of health that interest you. Reading, researching, and investigating can help spark creative ideas that you can implement in your family's lifestyle.

Find Support. Enlist your family, friends, or outside sources that encourage and lift you higher. Going through this change will not be easy. Having support can be essential to your success.

Give yourself a break! Be your own best friend. Love yourself into this transformation with the family. There will be mistakes, and that is OK! Remember, mistakes can be golden and direct you on the path you are supposed to be following. All parents and children make mistakes. We are all learning!

You can't change what you don't realize. If this is all new to you, do not be hard on yourself for not knowing the information beforehand.

Love yourself no matter what. Decide to take this journey with a massive amount of love, patience, and compassion for yourself and your children.

YOU set the tone for your family. Be a good role model. You don't have to do everything right to be a good role model. It's how you react in situations that make you a role model.

There is only one don't:

DON'T ever ever ever give up. You can do this! You and your child are worth every effort.

Guideline #5 What to Expect

The next five chapters in this Section consist of the Action Steps to help your child with their challenging behavior. Here is where the work begins! In Step 1, we will create a family blueprint by observing the current lifestyle. Step 2 has us laying a strong foundation by diving deep into nutrition and removing any foods that may be causing issues that affect your child. Continuing with nutrition in Step 3, we look at the quality and variety of meals and snacks. In Step 4, we build walls on our foundation with the areas of physical fitness, quality sleep and meditation, the mind, and the environment. Action steps are clearly laid out for you to pull all the areas of health together to make a solid structure and a healthy future. Take a deep breath, turn the page, and let's get started on the path to parenting the whole child!

Journal Points

What is your goal for this program?

What are you looking forward to the most?

Final Thought

Starting something new is easier than feeling the pain of staying stuck.

CHAPTER 10

STEP 1

MAKING A BLUEPRINT

With all the different categories of health to choose from, we must first start transforming your family's lifestyle, by looking into the area of nutrition for our solid foundation. Food is what fuels the body. It has an enormous effect on how we function and the quality of how our body feels. Food is the building block of how children behave and perform. Once the intake of food is of better quality and any sensitivities are eliminated, your child's behavior will naturally improve, and it will be easier to see if there are any other areas that are lacking. If you feel that there is more than one area your child needs help in, that is completely normal and more the case than not. In this chapter, we will dive into looking at how nutrition is affecting your child on a deeper level.

BECOME A DETECTIVE

As parents, we have to be flexible enough to take on different roles or switch hats, as I like to say, with our children. When our children are sick, we put on our doctor or nurse hat to see to it that they are cared for.

When our children have problems with their friends, we put on our counselor hat to listen and give advice as needed. When our children need help with their math homework we put on our teacher's hat. (Or in my case, I act as a principle to help direct them to their oldest brother who puts on his teacher's hat, for all math help.) In Step 1, we will be investigating the household lifestyle and for that.... we will need our detective hat. So, get it out and let's get to solving the behavior problem!

In order to make a blueprint, we must first start by making an observation of what is happening in the home. It's time to start wondering why your child behaves the way they do and uncover any hidden influences that have affected them by becoming a detective. Get curious, question, observe, investigate and start to do some of your own research. It is time to take what I call a whole life inventory. During this phase, you will only be observing and taking notes. You will look at the food eaten, the amount of quality sleep, physical fitness, behavior, moods, the environment and stress the child may feel. This is all discovery work. It is important not to attach too much emotion during this phase, especially if you tend to worry, be anxious or feel guilty. Instead, take a neutral observation of what is going on in your child's life. Keep in mind, we only know what we know at the time. Do not be hard on yourself and understand this process is to enhance and improve the whole family lifestyle. Step into your life with a different view. Leave the past behind and start a new journey. Enjoy the process of learning and discovery and enjoy learning together. No guilt attached! Let the learning begin!

SYMPTOMS CHECKLIST

Becoming aware of any issues can be hard to do if you do not know what you are looking for. In Chapter 4, there was a Symptoms Checklist provided. If you filled it out, now is the time to refer to it. If not, on the following page is the same checklist, which can help you discover where your child may or may not fit in. Becoming familiar with symptoms to look for, will help you navigate through Step 1. Symptoms are not limited to the checklist, so if your child has a symptom that is not listed, go ahead and write it down. The point of the checklist is for you to become aware and acknowledge any symptoms. The symptoms are not the problem though. The symptoms are the body telling you a story. Let's figure out what it's trying to say. This is important because it can help get you thinking about foods and how they can react with your child. This will give you a heads up to cue into certain foods and the common behaviors and reactions that can be caused by them. If you would like to print the Symptoms Checklist to add to your journal or binder, please visit my website at www.brittahelayne.com.

Symptoms Checklist

Ruling out sensitivities is important and can make a huge difference in a child's behavior. If you feel like your child may have a sensitivity reaction to food, but you are not sure what the food is, taking this Symptoms Checklist can help.

Does your child have symptoms of a food sensitivity? Circle or highlight the symptoms below that you feel your child exhibits. If there are symptoms that your child has that are not on the list, write them on the lines below.

Behavior- ADD/ADHD behavior (inattentiveness, hyperactive, lack of focus, restless), OCD behaviors (obsessive and repetitive behavior), irritability, poor eye contact, food cravings, poor comprehension, anger, brain fog, aggression, lack of interest, disorganized thinking and disorientation, anxiety, depression, moodiness, over emotional, inappropriate laughter

Circulatory System- elevated blood pressure, racing heart, irregular pulse

Digestive System- upset stomach, IBS, constipation, diarrhea, mucus in stool, nausea, vomiting, gas, cramping, heartburn, bloating, abdominal pain

General- fatigue, delayed growth, delayed puberty, lethargy, speech disorders, vision problems, cravings

Neurological System- headaches, migraines, dizziness, ears ringing, tics, insomnia, night terrors, sleep disruptions

Respiratory System- coughing, sore throat, clearing throat constantly, canker sores in the mouth, bleeding or swollen gums, tooth discoloration, excess mucus, runny nose, congestion, watery or itchy eyes, sinus problems, ear infections, nasal polyps

Skeletal and Muscular System- aches and pains, swelling, stiffness

Skin- dark circles under the eyes, rosy red cheeks and ears, acne, hair loss, skin disruptions and disorders, rashes, elbow rash, eczema, hives

Urinary System- edema, bladder infections

Others:

_____
_____
_____
_____
_____
_____
_____
_____

Common Offenders That Produce Symptoms

Any Sensitivity

Aches and Pains	Heartburn
Bloating	Irregular Pulse
Coughing	Irritability
Dark Circles Under Eyes	Racing Heart
Elevated Blood Pressure	Skin Rash and Hives
Fatigue	Swelling and Stiffness
Food Cravings	Throat Clearing
	Watery Itchy Eyes

Corn

ADD/ADHD Behavior	Lack of Concentration
Aggression	Lack of Focus
Anger	Moodiness
Anxiety	Night Terrors
Behavior Problems	OCD Behavior
Brain Fog	Skin Disruption and
Headaches	Disorders
Hyperactivity	Sleep Disruptions
	Tics

Dairy/Soy/Casein

Acne	Frequent Sinus Infections
Anxiety	IBS Constipation/Diarrhea
Behavioral Issues	Inappropriate Laughter
Brain Fog	Lack of Interest
Congestion	Mucus in Stools
Depression	Poor Comprehension
Eczema	Poor Eye Contact
Excess Mucus	Repetitive Behavior
Frequent Ear	Rosy Red Cheeks or Ears
Infections	Runny Nose
	Sore Throat

Gluten

ADD/ADHD	Eczema
Behavior	Elbow Rash
Anxiety	Frequent Bladder Infections
Bleeding or Swollen	Headaches
Gums	Inappropriate Laughter
Brain Fog	Lack of Interest
Canker Sores	Nausea
Constipation	Over Emotional/Moodiness
Cramping	Poor Comprehension
Delayed Growth	Poor Eye Contact
Delayed Puberty	Repetitive Behavior
Diarrhea	Tooth Discoloration
	Vomiting

Additives- Preservatives/Dyes/Flavor Enhancers/Fragrances

Abdominal Pain	Hyperactivity
Acne	Insomnia
Aggression	Lack of Concentration
Behavior Problems	Lack of Focus
Congestion	Lethargy
Disorganized Thinking	Migraines
Disorientation	Mood Swings
Dizziness	Nasal Polyps
Ear Infection	Nausea
Eczema	Ringing in Ears
Edema	Skin Rash
Gas	Speech Disorder
Headaches	Tics
Heartburn	Upset Stomach
Hives	Vision Problems

(Please note, symptoms can vary in each individual.)

JOURNAL

In the Introduction of this book, I asked you start a journal to answer Journal Points in the first two Sections. It is now time to add to the journal in a different way. During Step 1, it is important to keep a whole life inventory for one week. Keeping a Daily Health Journal Page will help paint a picture of what is currently going on in the household. It is crucial not to miss or skip this step of the process. The journal is something you will keep and look back on as a reference. In the future, you will see just how far your child has come. For the week, you will want to bring the journal everywhere you go, to get the most accurate descriptions. Journaling this way will allow you to pull all the areas of your child's life together. A whole life inventory will help figure out areas that need improvement and areas that are balanced. If you would like to print off the Journal Page, please visit my website at www.brittahelayne.com.

A few recommendations when journaling:

-It's ok to involve the family by having your child journal too. Not only will it help them practice writing, but it will also teach them to become more self-aware of what they are doing to their own bodies. This is SO important at any age!

-I suggested at the beginning of the book to use a binder with loose sheets of paper as your journal. Using a binder makes it easier to add pages.

-It is better to physically write down all the entries, rather than track everything on a computer or phone.

There are a few reasons for this. One is writing helps to promote better recall. Another reason is, at the end of this week, when the time comes to put all the entries together as a whole, you will be able to lay everything out in front of you and put the clues together.

-Be consistent. Do your best filling out an entire entry for the whole 7-day period. In the end, you will have a complete picture of what is going on in the household and a great reference book for your child.

-It's important at this stage that you do not change anything. Do the best you can to fill the journal out. Be honest and write everything truthfully and leave judgment behind, it has no place in your life!

-Making journal entries is not about blame, guilt, or who is doing what. There is no beating yourself up or being critical. It is about painting a picture of the present and deciding what to change to make your family healthy.

DAILY JOURNAL

A DAY IN THE LIFE OF_____

SLEEP	**EXERCISE**	**QUIET TIME**

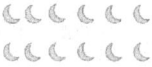

10 10 10
10 10 10

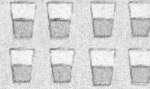

Awake: Asleep:

Daily Meals and Snacks

Time   Foods   Symptoms

WATER

ENVIRONMENT
STRESSORS

NOTES

_____

_____

_____

_____

CREATE A BLUEPRINT

Once you have your 7-day journal completed, decisions can be made about what type of actions need to take place. Layout the pages of the journal and the Symptoms Checklist and study them. Take an inventory of the information, so you can begin to see a pattern and an overall picture of your child's life. Next, write out any symptoms that you suspect have something to do with food. For instance, if you notice your child gets angry or whiny right before a meal, you could make a guess that perhaps the timing of meals affects your child's moods. Maybe you notice your child tantrums after they eat something with high fructose corn syrup, you can guess corn might be the problem. If your child gets hyperactive after they have eaten something with red dye, you can suspect additives to be the problem. Whatever you may suspect write it down. Do you see any correlations with food, mood, physical symptoms, and behavior?

After connecting some dots, think about what type of actions need to take place by deciding what food or foods your child may be sensitive to. Pick one highly suspectable food you would like to commit to eliminating in Step 2. If you do not feel as though any specific foods need to be avoided, I would advise you to allow some extra time to think about your child's symptoms and the checklist. If you still feel like no certain foods need to be avoided, go ahead and go to Step 2 and commit to picking more nutritiously dense selections of meals and snacks to serve your child.

Congratulations! You made a blueprint and you are done with Step 1. Make sure you take time to celebrate this success.

Journal Points

Symptoms Checklist

Daily Health Journal for 7 days

Final Thought

Being proactive is the best prevention of sickness, disease, and being unhealthy.

CHAPTER 11

STEP 2

LAY THE FOUNDATION

In Step 1, you journaled and started a discovery phase of what is currently going on in the home. You also committed to eliminating one food category, to see if improvement with your child's health and behavior take place. It is time to start following your unique blueprint using elimination and replacement. This is the start of your family's new lifestyle! There is a possibility, that when you begin changing current eating habits to healthier and safer choices, you may notice other areas of your child's life changing as well. Once you start cleaning up the diet, a domino effect can take place, changing the other aspects of health. Even though it may seem overwhelming at this moment to eliminate foods from the diet, get excited about the changes ahead that will make a difference in your child's behavior.

BECOME A COACH

Hopefully, you have started to see the connection between food and behavior. In Step 1, you put on a detective hat to investigate why your child behaves the way they do. In this Step, you will put on a coach's hat to begin the transformation of peeling away physical symptoms and bad behavior, to find your true child who may be masked by the foods they are eating. For the next three weeks, a process of elimination and replacement will take place. As a coach, you will guide and encourage your child to eat foods without ingredients you are wanting to avoid. In order to do this, you must become familiar with the ingredient or category you are eliminating and make a game plan for meals and snacks. Don't worry, I will be your coach to help you through this!

As a coach, it is extremely important that you use positive reinforcement during this process. You created a blueprint, now you will implement it with strategies I will lay out for you. Be a source of support for your family during this process. Change can seem hard but encourage everyone to stick with it and in the end, your family will come out as winners.

Trying new foods can be an adventure. No one has to like everything that is tried, but your child will start to discover that they may really like some foods they denied or didn't even know existed. Just like you would want your child to be a good sport when playing a game, expect them to be a good sport trying new foods. Again, they do not have to like everything, but the trying part... is huge! So, make sure you encourage participation and be creative! Let your kids know sitting on the sidelines watching isn't as fun as playing with the team.

Rules

It is important during this period that guidelines are in place. There are definite rules being the coach:

-Food is **never** taken away as a punishment.

-Do not be harsh on your child for not trying a new food or not liking something. Saying nothing is better than being negative.

-Involve the whole family and be a team.

-Be positive and supportive. Do not dread or talk negatively about foods and eating.

-It is important that you role model the behaviors you want to see.

-Being a coach means you are training and shaping leaders to become better versions of themselves by stretching and growing. Make sure you are doing the same!

GET TO KNOW WHAT WILL BE AVOIDED

Unless you are buying foods that are whole and in natural form without added ingredients, make sure you read the labels and become familiar with the names of the ingredients and what they consist of. Many foods have multiple names. If you are eliminating corn, you may not see the word corn listed in the ingredients. However, there are a large number of ingredients that have corn like dextrin's, glucose, and malt that you may not realize. If you are eliminating dairy, gluten, soy, corn or additives, I have provided common names associated with the ingredients in this Chapter and in the Appendix section of this book. Although the categories I have listed are common to cause symptoms, there are other foods that could be your child's culprit of issues that I did not include. If you are eliminating an ingredient other than what I have provided in this book, research and become familiar with the various names associated with it.

*Please note, in the section with Additives, there are too many additives to list. If an ingredient sounds like it has a chemical name, it most likely is a chemical. Make sure you research any ingredients you are unaware of.

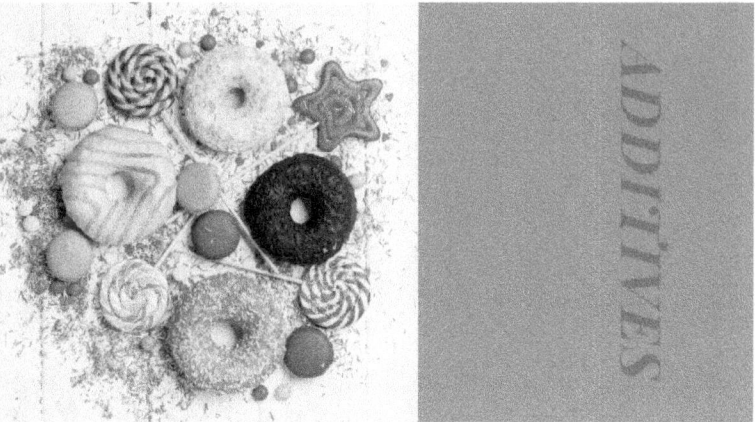

ADDITIVES

All Artificial food Coloring

All Artificial Sweeteners

BHA

BHT

BPA

Coloring

Fragrances

MSG

Nitrates

Nitrites

PFC

Perchlorate

TBHQ

If it sounds like a chemical, it probabaly is.

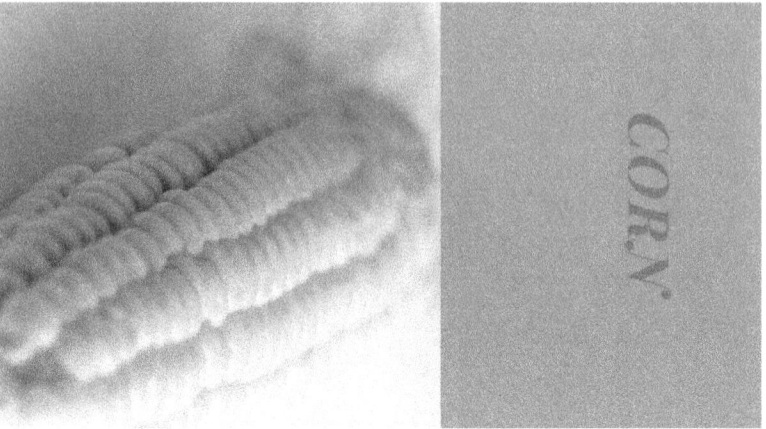

CORN

Alcohol
Artificial & Natural Flavors
Aspartame
Baking Powder
Bleached & Enriched Flour
Bleached & Enriched Sugar
Carmel & Carmel Coloring
Corn Starch
Flavoring
Food Starch
Cereal
Citric Acid
Confectioners Sugar
Anything with Corn
Crystalline Fructose
Dahlia Syrup
Dextrin & Dextrose
Erythritol
Folic Acid
Fructose
Glucose
Golden Syrup
Grits
Hominy
Hydrolyzed Protein

High Fructose Corn Syrup
Invert Sugar & Invert Syrup
Isoglucose
Lactic Acid
Lecithin
Maize
Malt
Maltitol
Maltodextrin
Mannitol
Modified Food Starch
MSG
Pectin
Polysorbate
Sorbitol
Starch
Vegetable Gum
Vinegar
Vitamin A
Vitamin C
Vitamin E
Xanthan Gum
Xylitol
Yeast
Zein

DAIRY

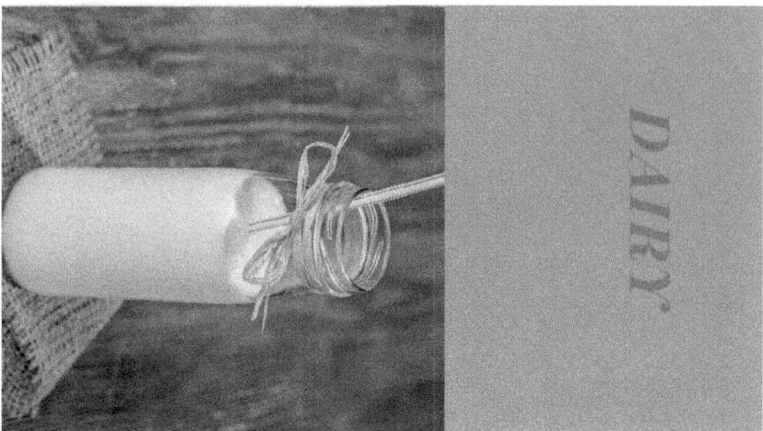

Artificial Butter and Flavor
Butter
Butter Extract
Buttermilk
Caesin
Caseinate
Cheese
Cheese Flavor
Condensed Milk
Cottage Cheese
Cream
Curds
Custard
Dry Milk
Evaporated Milk
Frozen Yogurt
Galactose
Ghee
Half and Half
Hydrolysates
Ice Cream
Kefir

Lactalbumin
Lactate Solids
Lactyc Yeast
Lactalbumin Phosphate
Lactoglobulin
Lactose
Lactulose
Milk
Milk Chocolate
Milk Solids
Nisin
Nougat
Pudding
Quark
Rennet
Sour Cream
Imitation Sour Cream
Whey
Whip Cream
Whipped Cream
Yogurt

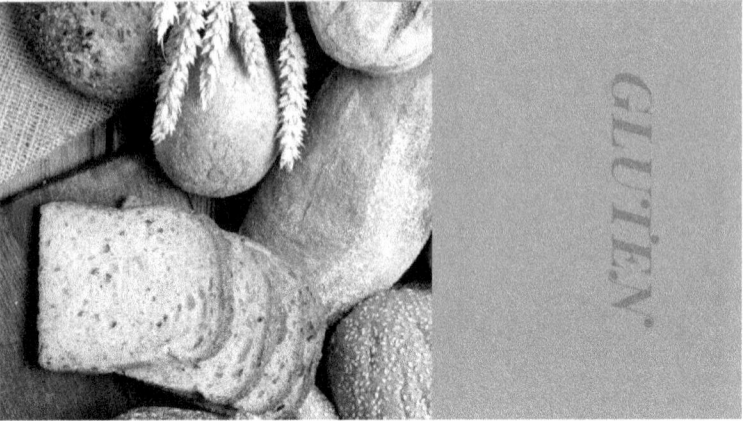

GLUTEN

All Purpose Flour
Atta
Barley
Brewer's Yeast
Bran
Bread
Bread Crumbs
Bulgar
Club Flour
Couscous
Cracker Meal
Durum
Eikorn
Emmer
Farina
Fu
Gluten
Graham Flour
Groats
Kamut
Maida
Malt
Matzo
Modified Food Starch

MSG
Natural Flavors
Noodles
Pasta
Oats
Rye
Seitan
Semolina
Spelt
Sprouted Wheat
Starch
Tabbouleh
Thickeners
Triticale
Triticum
Wheat
Wheat Berries
Wheat Bran
Wheat Germ
Wheat Grass
Wheat Protein Isolate
White Flour
Whole Meal Flour
Yeast Extract

120

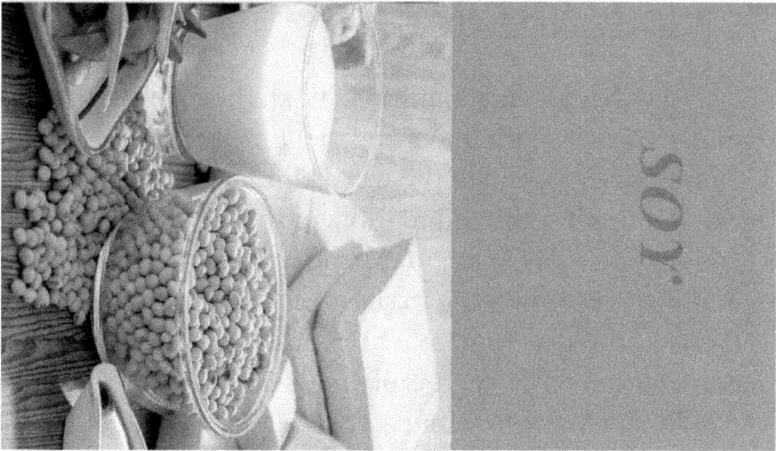

SOY

Artificial Flavors
Bean Curd
Edamame
Hydrolyzed Vegetable Protein
Kinako
Koya Dofu
Lecithin
Margarine
Mayonnaise
Miso
Mono & Diglycerides
Natto
Natural Flavors
Olean
Okara
Soy Formula
Soy Grits
Soy Lecithin
Soy Milk
Soy Miso
Soy Nuts
Soy Protein
Soy Protein Concentrate
Soy Protein Isolate
Soy Sauce
Soy Sprouts
Shoyu
Sobee
Soybean
Soybean Curds
Soybean Flour
Soybean Paste
Soya
Soya Flour
Tamari
Tempeh
Teriyaki Sauce
Tofu
Vegetable Broth
Vegetable Oil
Vegetable Shortening
Vegetable Starch
Vitamin E
Yuba

ELIMINATE AND REPLACE

Now that you are familiar with all the names of the food you are wanting to avoid, it's time to get eliminating! Although the word eliminate means to get rid of, I don't want you to think of this next process as taking food away from your family or child. This process is about experimenting to see what foods help and what foods hurt. Also, remember to stick to one category like corn, gluten or dairy. It is ok to have more than one you would like to try to eliminate, however, we will only begin with one. If two categories of food are eliminated at the same time and there is improvement, it will be hard to know which food is lessening the symptoms your child exhibits. Let's begin to take action against one offending food category by eliminating it and replacing it with something else.

Sensitivities to ingredients are not limited to food products. Make sure to check any vitamins being given or over the counter medications. Look at items applied topically such as creams, lotions, shampoo or sprays. The skin is the largest organ in the body and the body can still react sensitively to the ingredient even though it isn't being eaten. It's very important during this phase to avoid all things possible that the offending ingredients are in. Things can be added back at the end of the 3-week period, but they need to be completely avoided during that time to ensure that your child is as clean as possible from the offender.

Replace

For the next 3 weeks, you will replace the eliminated category with versions of food that do not contain the offending ingredient. By replacing foods, you can allow your inner creativity to shine. There are so many options today for food sensitivities. Let's start with an example of replacing dairy. There are a variety of cheeses, milk, butter, sour cream, ice cream and yogurt products made from nuts, oats, rice, soy, hemp, and coconut. When looking for a replacement, bring your checklist located in this Chapter and in the Appendix, to cross-reference with the ingredients on the product label. It is possible during this process that you see your child does very well with most dairy replacements but for some reason, with let's say a certain cheese replacement, obvious symptoms come back. Some dairy-free products still contain casein, which is a protein in milk that can wreak havoc on your child's body if they are sensitive to it. Study the ingredients, write them down or take a picture of them, and take this as another clue for the near future. In the meantime, avoid that certain product and try something else.

MAKE A MEAL AND SNACK PLAN

Making a weekly meal and snack plan and sticking to it, can be very helpful to your commitment to eliminate and replace. If you do not plan, it can be easy to feel overwhelmed. During this step, it is a great time to incorporate home cooking. If you like to cook, spectacular! If you do not, no worries, there are simple things you can do that will make you look like a Rockstar.

Ideas and a sample menu

-Use the internet to look for recipes that are free of the category you are trying to avoid, helping eliminate frustration. However, you can modify most recipes quite easily. When I first started to try to find recipes without corn, I thought it was nearly impossible. I soon learned to substitute things like cornstarch with a mixture of arrowroot and baking soda. I could use recipes I had or found and modify them easily. Yes, it's a little more work but your child is worth it.

-Enjoy the time cooking, even if it isn't your favorite thing to do. Be grateful and excited to try something new!

-Making big batches, instead of mixing for single-use, can be a time saver. Leftovers can be eaten or incorporated into another meal. This will save time and money. For instance, if I make chili one night, I may use the leftovers for part of the filling in a burrito for another dinner.

-Planning ahead for the week is extremely helpful and can help avoid many hours of wasted time a wondering what to eat, how to fix it and trips to the grocery store. If you are on a limited budget, planning is everything! Find recipes for items you already have in the pantry or refrigerator.

-Nutritious meals don't mean they have to be super expensive, but creativity certainly helps. Beans and rice are amazing fillers, and the most nutritiously dense versions are not very expensive! Eggs are inexpensive additions, as well as vegetables. Fresh organic vegetables can be inexpensive in comparison to canned or frozen vegetable. The taste of fresh food doesn't compare to canned or frozen versions.

-Pick new foods to try, but also show your child how to pick new foods and let them feel as though they are part of the team. Look through cooking magazines or take them to a grocery store. Let them help you cook and serve the family a new dish that they help create. Help them to encourage the family to eat new fun foods.

WEEKLY MENU

5-Day Meal and Snack Planner

MONDAY

BREAKFAST	Oatmeal with Wild Blueberries
LUNCH	Turkey Roll Up, Bean Chips with Salsa
DINNER	BBQ Chicken Stuffed Potato with Ranch Avocado Dip
SNACKS	Apple and Nut Butter/ Homemade Trail Mix

TUESDAY

BREAKFAST	Yogurt with Power Bites
LUNCH	Grilled Chicken Strips, Celery & Avocado Dip, Peaches
DINNER	Quesadillas
SNACKS	Crackers, Pepperoni &Cheese/Cinnamon Apples&Pecans

WEDNESDAY

BREAKFAST	Smoothie and Trail Mix
LUNCH	Lettuce Wraps, Kale Chips, Pickles and Orange Slices
DINNER	Tortilla Soup
SNACKS	Nuts and Grapes/Homemade french fries

THURSDAY

BREAKFAST	Eggs and Salsa
LUNCH	Salad with Garlic Bread
DINNER	Homemade Pizza and Pesto
SNACKS	Yogurt and Fruit/Date Rolls

FRIDAY

BREAKFAST	Banana Bread and Chicken Sausage
LUNCH	Leftover Pizza and Pineapple Rings
DINNER	Hamburgers with Roasted Sweet Potato Fries
SNACKS	Smoothie/Pretzels with Pesto

JOURNAL

Journaling once a day, at the end of the day, can be helpful to keep track of symptom reductions or ideas for what meals and snacks affected your child either positively or adversely. Refer to Chapter 10 in the journal section for help on how to keep a journal. A Journal page to print, is located in the Appendix of this book or on my website, www.brittahealyne.com.

STICK WITH IT

After you eliminate one category, it may take up to 3 weeks to see results. However, it is possible to see results immediately. This is where your patience will need to come in. Give this process time. Be kind to yourself. Becoming frustrated will not help and may hurt the process. If you need to, take a mini break. Go do something that is healthy and makes you happy. During this time period in my life, I did a lot of fiction reading that took my mind to another world, even if it was for 5 minutes. Reading was a way I could escape and take a complete break to refresh my mind and spirit. Find something that works for you! Maybe it's meditation, or using essential oils like lavender to calm, watch something that makes you laugh, or talk to a friend to blow off steam.

THE NEXT STEPS

If you see results within the 3-week time period, it's time to decide whether to eliminate another category or move on to Step 3 in Chapter 12. If you feel confident you have caught a sensitivity and are satisfied, move on. If you feel like several symptoms have been eliminated, but there is still something that isn't right, it is ok to move on or repeat Step 2 with another category of food.

When I was going through this transition with Benji and Braeden, I did a back to back elimination. I started with dairy and was very pleased to see results in a short amount of time. After that, I eliminated gluten and I noticed Braeden's behavior slightly improved, but something still wasn't right. I was frustrated because I saw improvement at times with gluten, but at other times he would completely act out. I stopped eliminating gluten and eliminated corn instead. That.... made all the difference in the world! Many gluten-free products contain corn, so I thought I was doing something good by going gluten free and in fact, I was giving him MORE corn than usual!

This process is not an exact science because everybody is different. Take your time in deciding to move forward, try another elimination or move on. At any time, if you feel like you missed something, you can always stop and go back a step. If you aren't sure what to do, move on and chances are when you add in the other steps in this book, you will become more in tune to your child and foods that affect them.

If you saw little to no results in symptoms during Step 2, ask yourself these questions:

Did you stick to the program of being free of the category for 3 weeks? Is there a hidden ingredient that is being overlooked in a product or products?

Look over the previous journaling and Symptoms Checklist. Decide if you should pick another category to eliminate and start with Step 2 again. If you do not feel as though you need to eliminate a category of food or ingredients, focus on giving your child a wider variety of foods, cooking meals at home, and using better-quality ingredients. Cleaning up these areas may trigger another area to improve so you can see the big picture clearly or have a better sense of what direction to go in.

Congratulations on making it through Step 2! In the Chapters ahead, we will dive into the quality of food, bedtime routines, aspects of the environment, as well as physical fitness. If you are ready, let's move on to start to build to the structure by adding in nutritious food and drinks and replacing unhealthy products with a healthier version.

Journal Points

Take time to look through your journaling again. Look back and assess the progress that has been made so far.

What have you learned?

What needs refining?

What are the symptoms your child is dealing with right now?

How are your child's moods?

Final Thought

Two steps down, two steps to go. You are halfway through the program!

CHAPTER 12

STEP 3

BUILD THE STRUCTURE

No one should ever feel like they are limited or without while we are making this lifestyle change. Feelings of what you can't have can promote unhealthy attachments to food, which is the opposite of what we want to do as parents. Our goal is to get our children eating healthy, so they feel the effects of a thriving body and not to suffer from unwanted behaviors or unpleasant physical side effects. In the next 14 days, we are going to concentrate on continuing to replace and adding fun new foods and dishes to the diet. It's time to make all the meals and snacks as healthy as possible! When I did this, I felt like I was on a quest to change my family's eating style from the average American diet to a healthy, cleaner nutritious diet. Sound hard? I promise you; it is easier to do than to live with a child feeling the effects of unhealthy foods.

REPLACING

If you have ever tried to stop a bad habit, you know just how challenging it can be. When we focus on a negative habit, often, it can become worse! You can feel controlled or tied to the pattern and feel like it is impossible to break. Instead of focusing on what you shouldn't do, if you focus on what you can do, the bad habit disappears. You will have replaced it!

If you have a bad habit of watching too much TV and would like to break it, you could make a list of everything you can do instead of watching TV. The list might include, reading a book, going out to dinner with a friend, writing in a journal, playing a game with your kids, preparing a meal for the next day, looking up new recipes to try, helping your kids with homework, working on a favorite hobby, and so on. There is an abundance of things you can do with your time instead of watching TV. Once you add those into your life, you won't want to watch TV because you will have replaced the time in other ways.

Just like with TV, we will apply this to your child's diet. Instead of focusing on what your child can't have, look at the possibilities they can have. If you want to cut down on the amount of sugar eaten, focus on the sweet vegetables and fruits you can add to the meal and snack plan. If you want to stop buying fast food, focus on finding fun new meals to try that are nutritious yet can be prepared quickly or ahead of time. In Step 3, we will begin to change habits by making meals and snacks better quality and more nutritious. Let's start by upgrading foods!

REPLACE WITH QUALITY

Replacing with quality food means to buy or make better selections of a product currently used with a healthier version. We will begin by going through your pantry and refrigerator to pick products that could use an upgrade. When I first started, ketchup was the first victim to receive a transformation. When the high fructose corn syrup version of the bottle of ketchup was half empty, I poured an organic version in with it. It looked like the same ketchup bottle to my children, but I was slowly changing the products by adding a better-quality version. Another product I switched was pancake syrup. Instead of using the version that has high fructose corn syrup in it, I replaced it with 100% maple syrup. My kids didn't notice or care as I did this! I continued replacing sugars, flours, bread, yogurts, and just about every food we had. I either swapped it with a better version, or I made my own. You can choose to transform your products all at once or in steps like I did. Doing it in stages is a slow introduction and can work well for picky taste buds.

There may be something your child will want to hang on to and not give up and that's ok. Workaround them and do not make a big deal about it. What you focus on will become front and center. If your child won't accept a healthy version of a food, go on and try something else. Come back to it at a different time.

I came up against a problem, with my second son, with only one product. One day, I walked into our living room, and there was a cereal intervention going on. What is a cereal intervention you ask? It's when you are ambushed by your children who want to discuss the new cereals you are buying. Jensen, the ringleader of the intervention, said to me, "We want our cereals back. We don't like the new cereals. They all taste bad! We NEED to have our old cereals back." Then he started listing which cereals he needed and why! It appeared I was dealing with junk cereal starved children! I held steady and kept trying different cereals. Back then, the choices were not as plentiful as they are these days. Well, I ended up winning 3 out of the four kids with the cereal battle. Jensen, I am sorry to say, never did come around. In fact, we still have cereal matches to this day, and he is STILL explaining why he doesn't like the cereals I buy. I haven't given up, though! I keep trying!

Over the next 14 days, look to see what you have in your refrigerator or pantry that you can start replacing with a healthier version. Remember, this doesn't have to be overwhelming or hard. Most of the process of replacing foods can be painless, minus any interventions your kids may have like my cereal one. The results will be huge and can be very dramatic! Small steps can add up to equal significant changes! You cannot expect to replace everything overnight or even in the 14 days. The point is to start to get into the habit that will carry through to a new sustainable healthy lifestyle. Six months from now, you may still be replacing things, and that's totally ok!!! Take the time and do it right.

ADD MORE VARIETY

I once heard a doctor talking about how he tries to incorporate at least 20 different fruits and vegetables in his diet per day. Although this may sound impossible to you, it's a good guideline to use to see how many different fruits and vegetables you can add to meals and snacks every day. I use this as a guideline when I plan my meals for the week. Here's what it might look like: I always eat at least one salad a day, because I love salads! So, I may have spinach, kale, romaine lettuce, carrots, purple onions, parsley, and cucumbers as part of my salad for one meal. That's seven different sources of nutrients at one sitting. Another meal I may have is Tortilla Soup, which contains vegetable broth, green peppers, white onions, garlic, cilantro, tomatoes, corn, and it's topped with avocado and lime. You can see a variety of fruits and vegetables can add up throughout the day with little effort. In this section, I have listed many ideas of how you can incorporate fruits and vegetables into your family's meals and snacks. Give it your best shot and see how many of the ideas you can incorporate for the next 14 days. Come up with your own ideas and write them down in the space provided or add them to your journal.

Ideas for Variety

-Incorporate different fruits and vegetables weekly, other than what you have eaten the week before. It is so easy to get stuck eating the same thing over and over. Try to avoid this! Choose a variety by eating a rainbow of different colors. Eating this way will help your family benefit from the different nutrients offered.

-Preparing fruits and vegetables in different styles can be a fun way to mix things up a bit. If your child likes carrots, you can serve them raw, roasted, steamed, or sautéed. You can dice them, shred them, cut them in sticks, or cut them in coin sizes.

-Add toppings to your meals. If you have hamburgers one night for dinner, try adding vegetable toppings so the kids can pick out what they want on their burgers. If you have super picky children that will not try anything, you can offer it anyway and set a good example of eating the vegetables on your burger without making a big deal about them picking nothing. Talk about the toppings add a delicious flavor to a plain hamburger. Setting an example of good healthy eating habits can go a long way.

-Add in vegetables and herbs to your meals. A few examples could be making burritos with fresh cilantro, green peppers, and tomatoes, making hamburgers patties mixed with chopped spinach and tomatoes, or roasting homemade french fries with rosemary and olive oil.

-Pureeing food to add to the mixtures is a sneaky way to add nutrients for a picky child. For example, make homemade spaghetti sauce and add in pureed green vegetables. If you do not have time to make a homemade sauce, use a jar sauce and add in fresh garlic, onions, oregano, basil, pureed carrots, and pureed spinach.

-Make homemade pesto's with ingredients like garlic, olive oil, pine nuts, sun-dried tomatoes, and basil. These are delicious on pizzas, crackers, toppings for chicken, the possibilities are endless!

-Make a fruit salad with fresh fruits adding in one new fruit that the child hasn't tried.

-Make trail mix adding in a new nut or dried fruit like mulberries or coconut.

Add your own ideas:

_____

_____

_____

_____

_____

HAVE FUN

YOU have done an amazing job to get to this point. I understand all the pain and frustration you have felt before and even during this process. Take some time and have fun! Make sure you aren't taking everything too seriously, which can be easy to do when stressed. Watch a funny movie, relive fun memories with family or friends, call someone that is a ray of sunshine, get around positive people, or watch clips of your favorite scenes in movies. You could even put your headphones on and listen to your favorite music! Although, if you have kids in the house, keep one headphone out of your ear... I say this from the experience of having four boys. (Having both headphones in my ears listening to music,

set me up to be oblivious to pranks... hearing *nothing.)
No matter what you do, take a fun break, and enjoy
where you are, who you are, and your family.

Congratulations on making it through Step 3! Your
commitment and hard work are nothing short of
amazing! In Chapter 13, we will continue to design our
healthy family lifestyle by building the walls on our
strong foundation of nutrition, with the other aspects of
health.

Journal Points

What foods can you transform to a healthier version?

What are some ideas you have about adding more variety to your family's meals?

Final Thought

Walk your talk and be consistent.

CHAPTER 13

STEP 4

PUTTING IT ALL TOGETHER

Steps 1-3 of this program concentrated on turning bad behaviors around using better nutrition. In the next part of the journey, we will look at the other areas of heath and implement healthier actions for your child's everyday life. As we did with nutrition, we must first assess the different aspects of health to decide where to start, set a goal, and implement a plan to achieve the desired outcome. Put on your detective hat one more time, and let's get busy with Step 4!

SOWING SEEDS

In Section 2, we talked about five different areas of health, including nutrition, physical fitness, sleep and meditation, the mind, and the environment. Now we're going to ask ourselves specific questions in each of those categories to see how we can improve. Before we do that, I would like to paint a picture with an example of how we will tackle each area, the questions we will ask, and the action steps we will take to achieve the goals.

As I'm currently writing to you, I'm sitting at my kitchen table looking outside at my front yard. Unfortunately, I had two trees die recently. I was so sad and bummed because I liked the trees in my yard! I live in the Arizona desert and during the summer, it gets blazing hot. The trees were mature and offered a lot of shade, which is hard to come by. The trees died in the middle of summer, all the leaves fell, and I didn't get the shade that the trees once provided.

I held out for a long time, passed the time that I should of before the trees were cut down. I hung on to the idea that if I kept watering the trees, they would come back to life. I didn't want to let go, even though I knew that the outlook of the trees was dismal. My front yard looked unhealthy, but I held on hoping that if I kept doing the same thing that I was doing, I would see a spark of life. I waited until the trees were dead and dry before I had them cut down, which I do not recommend! I made a goal to redo my front yard. I wanted it to look prettier than before with a heartier kind of tree that would offer the shade I needed.

To meet my goal, first, I identified the trees were dead, and it was time to do something about them. Next, I had to implement steps or a plan to redo my yard, starting with cutting down the dead trees. Then, I needed to go to a garden store to pick out a new type of tree, flowers, and shrubs that I wanted in my yard. Once I bought and brought them home, I placed them precisely where I wanted them planted. The first time I arranged them, I did not like how I placed them. I started over and arranged the plants in a more pleasing way that worked for my yard and that I enjoyed. After that, a landscaper came out to plant them. Now they're all planted beautifully, and I love the way my front yard looks!

The plants and the tree are small and require water often. If I don't water them every day, they will start to wither and look unhappy. I can't instantly make them grow, although I would really like that because they aren't at the height I want them to be. However, if I take care of them properly and water them consistently, a year from now, my yard will look so much better! My shrubs will be bigger, and I will have more privacy. The flowering plants will be fuller and have more blooms. My baby tree will be a medium-size tree that will have more shade cover then it has now.

If you apply that whole scenario of my front yard to a situation of everyday life, it will take those same sets of actions to meet any health goals. Planning, deciding, implementing, watering, and consistency are the actions that must take place for change. Sometimes we hang on to things even though we know that it isn't healthy or the best thing to do. We hold out and hope something will change, although we didn't bring anything new into the situation to make the change. Often, it's best to clean the slate and start over fresh and healthy. This principle is just what we will practice in Step 4.

CREATE THE CHANGE

In this Chapter, I will list the five categories of health. I will ask you a few specific questions that will require you to be thoughtful, thorough, and investigate each category to make your family's lifestyle healthier. After you answer the questions, you will pick one category to start with and improve. As we've discussed before, beginning with one category, one goal, and taking small steps will lead to success. Anything more can be too overwhelming and can ultimately be a set up for failure.

In the past, I have put a time limit as a guide for each Step. However, this is the final Step of this process, where there is no time limit. In fact, you will be practicing this Step from here on out. Step 4 is about creating balance with all the health categories. Finding balance is an ongoing process in life and should be something we all strive to do. When balancing an area, you will continually adjust to fit the needs of your growing child and family.

For each set of questions in the categories, I have included examples to help you understand what the answers may look like. Read through the examples and come up with your solutions to fit your family. It's ok to read ahead to the next chapter, before you start answering questions. Chapter 14 is a Special Help guide that may be used as a reference. It lists all the different health categories with ideas and scenarios to help you create goals and action steps for change.

Create the Change

For each different category of health, answer the set of questions to help layout the obstacle, solution, goal, and action steps. Take your time and answer each question using details.

Example of a general answer and a detailed answer:

General response: *I would like a yard that is healthy and pretty.*

Detailed response: *I would like a tree in my yard to provide a large area of shade, shrubs that grow large enough to serve as privacy for my windows, and flowering plants placed all over to create colorful bursts of beauty.*

Examples of answers are listed for all the questions in each category. If more help is needed, refer to Chapter 14, Special Help. This activity is also in the Appendix of this book. If you would like to print the pages off, please go to my Website, www.brittahclaync.com.

Nutrition *Example*

Pick one to three different areas of nutrition you would like to see the most significant change. For each one, answer the following questions:

What would you like to change most about nutrition for your child?

I want my child to eat less starchy carbs for snacks in the form of crackers, bars, and chips and have him eat more fruits and vegetables.

I want to cook more dinners and snacks from scratch using fresh ingredients and herbs and spices.

I want to try to add more variety to my meals. I find myself using the same recipes over and over.

Which of those changes would you like to start with first, and why?

I want to start with my child eating more fruits and vegetables for snacks because I feel like this is the place where I can make the biggest impact for him to get more vitamins and minerals his growing body needs.

If you had that in place, what would the end goal look like?

Snacks would be a variety of fresh whole fruits and vegetables. My kitchen would be stocked with fresh foods instead of boxes and bags of prepared foods. Snacks will be well balanced and nutritiously dense.

After meeting the goal, how would you and your child feel? What would this mean for your family?

I would feel like my child was getting more natural nutritionally complete foods full of vitamins and minerals. My child would feel healthier, more energetic, and have a higher self-outlook about his body, eating fresh whole fruits and vegetables. Eating this way would save money on wasted produce and buying snacks that are boxed and higher priced.

What are the steps you can take to create that change?

1. I will have my child help pick out fruits and vegetables at the grocery store or farmer's market.

2. I will make ready-made snack trays that include his selections of fresh fruit and vegetables and a starchy carb, so he has a little of what he wants while getting fresh produce.

3. I will add nutritious dips made with fresh produce and herbs, so he is eating double the amount of fresh fruits and vegetables.

Nutrition

Pick one to three different areas of nutrition you would like to see the most significant change. For each one, answer the following questions:

What would you like to change most about nutrition for your child?

Which of those changes would you like to start with first, and why?

If you had that in place, what would the end goal look like?

After meeting the goal, how would you and your child feel? What would that mean for your family?

What are the steps you can take to create that change?

Physical Fitness *Example*

Pick one to three different areas of physical fitness, you would like to see the most significant change. For each one, answer the following questions:

What would you like to change most about physical fitness for your child?

My children spend too much time playing on their phones and not enough time being physically active.

I want my children to take more of an interest in exercising to help them stay fit, flexible, and injury-free.

Which of those changes would you like to start with first, and why?

I want my children to take more interest in physical fitness in their life so they will have healthier bodies.

If you had that in place, what would the end goal look like?

My children would be getting at least 60 minutes thorough out the day of exercise. They would be physically fit, ready to take on adventures such as hiking, camping, or other activities that require endurance that they would like to try and not have to worry about injuries, lack of health, incoordination.

After meeting the goal, how would you and your child feel? What would this mean for your family?

My child would feel strong, capable, and more confident, knowing they have strength and endurance. We could do activities together that would create opportunities to bond with one another.

What are the steps you can take to create that change?

1. Together, we will choose an activity the whole family can participate in as a goal, such as hiking on a 5-mile trail. We will research places hike and decide when and where to go on our family outing.

2. We will determine what exercises to do, to get in shape for a hike and how often to exercise.

3. I will make a chart to list out the exercises that each of us can post and follow.

4. We will each do those exercises for a reasonable amount of time weekly.

5. On the decided date, we will go on the 5-mile hike.

Physical Fitness

Pick one to three different areas of physical fitness you would like to see the most significant change. For each one, answer the following questions:

What would you like to change most about physical fitness for your child?

Which of those changes would you like to start with first, and why?

If you had that in place, what would the end goal look like?

After meeting the goal, how would you and your child feel? What would that mean for your family?

What are the steps you can take to create that change?

Sleep and Meditation *Example*

What would you like to change most about sleep and meditation for your child?

I have a teenager that stays up too late at night and is not getting the amount of sleep his body needs. The lack of sleep is affecting his moods and his performance in school.

I want to help my child learn a meditation, but I don't know how to begin.

My children have no set bedtime routine. Some nights they are up until midnight. My husband and I are always tired the next day. We can't seem to get a handle on the problem.

Which of those changes would you like to start with first, and why?

I want to teach my child to meditate, so when he gets upset, he will have something to help him calm himself immediately.

If you had that in place, what would the end goal look like?

My child would be able to control his emotions and catch himself before he gets out of control. Ultimately, he will be able to feel himself when he starts to get upset and know what to do to calm down.

After meeting the goal, how would you and your child feel? What would that mean for your family?

My child would feel less stressed out and overwhelmed and be able to handle tough situations in a better way.

I would feel relieved and happy that I was able to teach something my child can carry into the future. Together, we could all learn the skills to become more peaceful individuals, which will positively affect our family dynamics.

What are the steps you can take to create that change?

1. Research and choose a few meditations that I would like to try with my child.

2. I will ask my child which meditation he would like to try.

3. I will create a special meditation corner that any family member can go to if they are feeling upset, stressed, or out of control.

4. My child and I will decorate the corner. We will put a few snacks, water bottles, books, a soft blanket, and a pillow in the area.

5. We will practice the specific meditation, and I will make a laminated sheet to follow as a guide.

Sleep and Meditation

Pick one to three different areas of sleep and meditation you would like to see the most significant change. For each one, answer the following questions:

What would you like to change most about sleep and meditation for your child?

Which of those changes would you like to start with first, and why?

If you had that in place, what would the end goal look like?

After meeting the goal, how would you and your child feel? What would that mean for your family?

What are the steps you can take to create that change?

The Mind *Example*

What would you like to change most about the mind for your child?

My child has low self-confidence. She won't try anything new because she feels as though she won't be able to do the activity.

My child keeps saying he is stupid and not good at reading.

My child is hanging around friends that aren't the best influence. I feel like this is because he has a low self-outlook about himself.

Which of those changes would you like to start with first, and why?

I want to help my child stop saying he's stupid and not good at reading. I don't want him to grow up thinking he can't learn. Thinking this way, gives him a negative outlook about himself.

If you had that in place, what would the end goal look like?

He would feel confident when reading and be able to read and comprehend the information. He would have a favorable view about himself.

How would you and your child feel after the goal was met? What would that mean for your family?

My child would have more confidence in himself and his schoolwork. He would be a friend to himself, thinking thoughts such as I can do anything, I put my mind to.

What are the steps you can take to create that change?

1. *Today, we will sit down and talk to see what he is interested in reading. I will assure him; reading involves practicing and I'll use an example of another time in his life that required practice.*

2. *I will buy or print off stories or articles that my child might like to read.*

3. *Today I will read to him, take turns reading, or have him read, without making him feel pressured to perform.*

4. *I will commit to a time to read with him. Practice reading with him at least 10 minutes a day 3-5 times a week.*

The Mind

Pick one to three different areas of the mind you would like to see the most significant change. For each one, answer the following questions:

What would you like to change most about the mind for your child?

Which of those changes would you like to start with first, and why?

If you had that in place, what would the end goal look like?

After meeting the goal, how would you and your child feel? What would that mean for your family?

What are the steps you can take to create that change?

The Environment *Example*

What would you like to change most about the environment for your child?

I use store-bought cleaners with chemicals, and I would like to learn how to make my own to save money and create a less toxic environment for my family.

My child's room is a mess. I would like to have an organization system in place.

The refrigerator in the kitchen needs to be cleaned out. It is always hard to find anything in it.

My house is a mess, and every room seems unorganized and cluttered.

Which of those changes would you like to start with first, and why?

I want to clean the whole house. It's cluttered, unorganized, and just a mess. Every time I look around, I get discouraged.

If you had that in place, what would the end goal look like?

Each room in the house would have a great feel to it. I would be able to get other work done and spend time with the family, instead of continually trying to clean up little messes made days ago. Everything would have a place in our home.

After meeting the goal, how would you and your child feel? What would that mean for your family?

My family and I would be proud to have an organized home. We could concentrate on everyday living and not get stressed with an unorganized house. After clearing out the clutter and putting items where they belong, we wouldn't waste so much time looking for things we misplace.

What are the steps you can take to create that change?

1. Decide on one area or room to start organizing.

2. Get four boxes, one for trash, one for donating, one to give away, and one for a future yard sale.

3. Commit to at least 30 minutes per day of work, until the room is organized.

4. Assign family members to a task in each room.

The Environment

Pick one to three different areas of the environment you would like to see the most significant change. For each one, answer the following questions:

What would you like to change most about the environment for your child?

Which of those changes would you like to start with first, and why?

If you had that in place, what would the end goal look like?

After meeting the goal, how would you and your child feel? What would that mean for your family?

What are the steps you can take to create that change?

Journal Points

Create the Change

Final Thought

You are all the inspiration your child needs.

CHAPTER 14

SPECIAL HELP

THE WHOLE CHILD REFERENCE

This Chapter can be used as a reference to help work through the obstacles, goals and solutions for the Create the Change activity in Chapter 13. In this Chapter, I lay out specific actions of the five categories of health that make up the whole child. Each category has ideas to help you upgrade to healthier habits. You may read the five different sections in order or choose to skip around according to your child and family needs.

NUTRITION

Most of this book so far has covered the right nutrition for your child and the tremendous impact it has on behavior and overall wellbeing. We have spent a lot of time cleaning up the diet. We will continue to round out the category of nutrition by looking at cooking at home, adding herbs, and drinking more water.

Home-cooking

Cooking and eating meals at home will not only save money, but it's a healthier way to eat in general. Here are a few tips you can use to help make cooking at home a more manageable and cost-effective process:

-Short on time? Meal prepping for a few days or a week can help save time, money, and ensure your family is eating healthy meals and snacks.

-Don't let fresh produce go to waste! You can prepare fruits and vegetables ahead of time by chopping or prepping them for future meals. Freezing unused portions will save you money in the long run. Frozen fruits and vegetables also make great additions to smoothies!

-Don't leave home without a snack. Take the time to prepare snacks at home that can be taken with, on the go. Does your snack need to be refrigerated? No problem! Put the snacks in a small cooler or lunch bag with a cold pack.

-Make your own nutritious broths and stocks by using leftover vegetables and meats.

Vegetable Broth- Fill a large stock pot with any vegetables and herbs. Let it simmer for at least 4 hours. *Chicken or Turkey Broth*- Put a whole turkey or chicken in a large stock pot and cover with water. Add any desired vegetables or herbs. Let it simmer for at least 4 hours. *Chicken or Turkey Stock*- Put leftover chicken or turkey bones in a large stock pot and fill with water. Add in any vegetables, herbs and spices. Let simmer for up to 24 hours.

Flavor with fresh herbs

Need a different way to add flavor to meals? Add fresh herbs! Cooking with fresh herbs is a great way to upgrade your meals. Herbs have medicinal properties, so while you may be using them to add flavor to your dishes, they can also be used as a medicine to treat and keep health in balance.

Here are a few of my favorites and how you can use them for your family's health:

Parsley is a chelator, which helps remove heavy metals in the body. It binds with the metals and removes the toxins out of the body. Parsley is also a diuretic, helping to eliminate water retention. Use parsley in smoothies, salads, meat mixtures, casseroles, soups, and dips.

Cilantro has many benefits for the body. It is high in antioxidants which help keep cells in the body from being damaged. Like parsley, it chelates heavy metals. Cilantro also helps lower blood sugar, prevent urinary tract infections, and can even lower anxiety levels. Cilantro is excellent for Mexican dishes, salsas, sauces, and soups.

Garlic is a great addition that can be used to kill bacteria, viruses, yeasts, and parasites in the body. Garlic is great for balancing blood sugar and keeping the heart healthy. Use garlic for roasting, sautéing, vegetables and meat dishes, casseroles, and in salads.

Rosemary has therapeutic properties and is an excellent help for cold and flu viruses. Rosemary is also stimulating to the brain and energizing to the body. Add rosemary to vegetable dishes, soups, meat dishes, or to flavor water.

Thyme can be used to cleanse the body. It is excellent to use against any viruses. It can help with any congestion, working as an expectorant. Use thyme to drink in hot water for illnesses, as flavoring to soups, stews, and meat dishes.

Oregano can help chase away any bacteria or viruses in the body. It is great to use for any respiratory illnesses, helping to open the lungs. Oregano is a powerful way to kill candida in the body. Use oregano in Italian dishes, soups, stews, and to flavor hot water to drink for medicinal purposes.

Marjoram is used to help relax respiratory conditions, help with digestive issues such as gas, and as a pain killer. Use marjoram in soups, salads, and meat dishes.

Lemon Grass has many benefits, such as eradicating candida, reducing acne, and as a pain killer. Use to flavor hot or cold water, in steam for the face, desserts, Asian Dishes, soups, and sauces.

Drink more water

Is your child complaining about drinking plain water? Water doesn't have to be boring! Here is a way to help encourage your child to drink more water by adding flavor:

Get a mason or a glass jar, add water, and your favorite choices from the list below. Refrigerate the filled jar for a few hours or overnight, depending on how strong you would like the flavor. Before long, your child will have a drink that tastes and looks refreshing! Serve it to your child in a special cup or water bottle.

Infuse water with flavor:

Fruit- lemon, strawberries, orange, lime, grapefruit, mango, kiwi, watermelon, apple, honeydew, blueberries, raspberries, blackberries

Vegetables-carrots, cucumber, sweet peppers

Herbs- mint, rosemary, lemongrass

Spices- cinnamon stick, vanilla bean, fennel, basil, anise

PHYSICAL FITNESS

In Chapter 5, I discussed why physical activity is crucial to children of all ages. There are no cookie-cutter exercises for a one size fits all program. Help your child find an activity that exercises their body, challenges them, and, most importantly, they enjoy. The activity can be varied and doesn't have to be the same thing over and over. Incorporating exercise doesn't have to take up a lot of time and can be added throughout the day. Five minutes here and there can really add up! The goal is to get your child moving and understanding, no matter the age, fitness is essential to life every day.

Examples of incorporating fitness into an everyday routine:

Every night before bed, take 5 or 10 minutes to do stretching or Yoga.

After waking do 5 or 10 minutes of stretching or Yoga.

Walk to the bus stop.

Ride a bike to school.

Have your child ride their bike to a friend's house instead of getting a ride.

Take the stairs instead of riding in an elevator or on an escalator.

Walk the dog.

Park further away in the parking lot to add extra steps.

After watching TV for a ½ hour, plan a 10-minute exercise break for everyone.

Family walk after dinner.

Hike in nature.

Walk to a store or restaurant, if the area permits.

Stop at a park to play and walk around.

When traveling, pack meals and stop at parks for a 20-minute break to get out and exercise.

Make an obstacle course or have your child make an obstacle course.

On a hot or cold day, go to a mall and walk around.

Take everyone geocaching.

Sprint while keeping track of times.

Create an exercise routine to a favorite or funny song.

Hula Hoop to music.

Play catch with your kids.

Go fishing.

Research and try a new sport.

Have a dance contest.

Play a game of darts.

Toss beanbags in buckets.

Join a walkathon as a family and design exercises to get everyone ready.

Have everyone list a goal for the month to exercise and create plans to help meet the goal.

Keep track of steps with a step counter. Whoever wins gets to pick a movie, plan the next activity, make their favorite meal, or pick a favorite board game to play.

It might seem like many of the activities listed are for younger children. However, this is not the case! Teens need to feel included and part of the family. It is essential! If they do not get it from their family, they will look elsewhere. So, include them, even if they act like it's the worst thing in the world. Keep including them and make it mandatory. For instance, Let's say you decide to go to the zoo for a day of bonding with the family and exercise. Don't give your children of any age a choice not to go. I don't pretend to think all outings or family activities are "fun" for everyone, especially if there is a teen attitude involved. Children, especially teens, do a lot of acting like they don't want or need anything. During these years, they need you just as much as when they were younger.

SLEEP

Bedtime needs to be a pleasant way to end the day, not an exhausting, chaotic ritual that leaves you and your child stressed out, burned out, and angry. Here are suggestions to ensure a quality night's rest:

Keep a bedtime routine

One of the best things you can do to set your child up for good quality sleep is to stick to a bedtime routine. When you have a nightly routine, the body naturally knows what to do at bedtime. Children crave and want a schedule. Having a plan helps your child understand what to expect and how to do each bedtime task.

No matter the age of your child, you create the atmosphere around bedtime. Being part of a bedtime routine is an excellent way to connect with your child. During the teen years, when they are oh so busy, this can be one thing to count on for a few precious moments of connection. Make sure no matter what has happened that day, you find them, hug them, and tell them how proud you are of them. Never miss an opportunity to discuss with your child how much you love them and how happy you are that you are their parent. What an amazing way to end each night, making your child feel loved and secure!

Example of a bedtime routines

5:00 Dinner and clean up	7:30 Clean up for 10 minutes
6:15 Playtime outside	7:40 Get ready for the next day (pack backpack, lay out clothes, pack lunch)
7:00 Small snack	
7:30 Bath time, brush teeth and PJ's on	8:00 Stretching
8:00 Read books	8:20 PJ's on and brush teeth
8:30 Say good night and lights out	8:45 Read book
	9:15 Lights out, say goodnight, and use meditation

Write out a schedule you would like to implement with your child. Make sure it is reasonable and not too overwhelming. A schedule must include enough activity for the child's body to recognize that it is nighttime. Each night try to stick to it as close as you can without distraction. If something about the schedule doesn't work, change it! It is all up to you. Do what works best for you and your child.

Sunlight

What does sunlight have to do with sleep? Sun aids in the production of a hormone called melatonin, produced by the pituitary in the brain. Melatonin is the hormone that stimulates sleep. Without enough melatonin in the body, it will be hard to fall asleep and stay asleep. To ensure a good night's rest, it starts way before it is bedtime. Make sure your child gets enough fresh air and sun during the daytime hours.

Winding down

It's essential to help your child's body wind down at night. Going to bed right after vigorous exercise, a dramatic movie, a large meal, or a stressful event can be hard for your child to do. Sending the body signals that it is time to wind down can help prepare your child for a goodnight's rest.

Sometimes, getting the body to relax can be a challenge. Here are a few ways to help signal the body it's time to relax and quiet down:

Stretching

Yoga poses

Read

Write in a journal

Drawing in a journal

Tell your child a story/child tells a story

Put away toys for the day

Say goodnight to pets or favorite stuffed animal

Eating

Eating shortly before bedtime can keep your child up at night. It can also cause your child to wake up during the night. Nighttime is the way the body recovers before going to sleep. If the body is busy trying to digest, it will use up precious time to digest instead of recover and rest.

Caffeine

Some caffeine is naturally occurring in foods such as dark chocolate, coffee, or tea. However, adding caffeine to the diet can be troublesome when it comes to getting sleep. Caffeine is a stimulant that affects the brain and the heart. Even having small amounts during the day can keep your child from falling asleep and staying asleep at night. If your child does have caffeine, limit it to daytime only.

Additional Ideas

If you still feel like your child has a hard time calming down before bed, try these tips:

Diffuse lavender essential oil.

At bath time, add in Epsom Salts and lavender to the water.

Read to your child. Your child is never too old to have a story read to them.

Sing a special song to them or with them every night.

Try Flower Remedies for a gentle way to help relax the body.

Consider a white noise machine.

Use a dim side table lamp in your child's room at night instead of bright overhead light.

Leave all negative emotions outside the bedroom. Don't bring emotions like anger, anxiety, fear or stress as the night winds down.

Add tart cherries juice to the diet.

Vitamins and supplements that may help your child- Magnesium, Potassium, Melatonin, Omega 3, Calcium, Vitamin B, and 5- HTP.

Essential Oils that may aid in sleep- Lavender, Jasmine, Lemon Balm and Valerian.

MEDITATION

A fantastic way to get the mind and body to relax is meditation. If your child has a difficult time calming down, any of these meditations can be very helpful.

Relaxing Movements

Yoga- helps to balance and relax the body. Try Easy Pose, Butterfly Pose, Corpse Pose, Cat Pose and Childs Pose

Static Stretching- stretching signals the muscles to relax. Try stretches from head to toe

Belly Breathing

Have your child lay down and put one hand on their stomach and the other hand over their heart. Have them breathe in through the nose and inflate their stomach like a balloon. Then, exhale out of the mouth slowly, letting all the air out of their stomach like a deflating balloon.

Visualization

There are many ways you can use visualization as a meditation. The idea is to get your child to a relaxed state by thinking calming happy thoughts. You might suggest that your child imagines themselves at a time when they were happy or in a calming place like a beach or forest.

Guided meditation

If your child has a difficult time calming down to meditate, this may be the best type of meditation to use. There are specialized apps that can be used for your child to listen to a meditation. If you choose, you may record your voice and guide your child through a meditation. It can be as simple as slowly and quietly talking them through relaxing parts of the body starting from the toes ending at the top of their head. Example: Relax the toes, feet, ankles, legs, waist, chest, fingers, wrists, hands, arms, shoulders, neck, mouth, eyes, and head.

THE MIND

The earlier we teach our children having a healthy mind is crucial to wellbeing, the better off they will be.

Here are a few ways you can direct your child and make a big difference in their outlook of everyday life:

Habits

Giving up can be easy for anyone, especially if you are waiting for a change to happen, and you don't see instant results. Neuroscience studies show, that it takes 30 days to make or break a habit. It is easier to replace a habit rather than break one. Never focus on a bad habit. Whatever is focused on grows, so make sure you are emphasizing the positive.

Examples:

If your child is overeating sugar, focus on eating nutritious meals by adding more sweet vegetables and protein, or focus on replacing the sugar with fruit.

If your child plays too many video games, focus on interacting with your child. You could play a card or board game, go outside and play catch, or ride bikes together.

If your child is doing poorly in a subject at school instead of focusing on what they are doing wrong, focus on what they can learn to improve. Take the time to sit down and see what the specific problem is. Focus on helping and practicing skills.

All these scenarios will take time to overcome. There is no quick fix to address these obstacles! Small situations of everyday life are chances to teach your child good practices. You can make a giant impact on your child's brain and self-esteem. Teaching them good habits is something they will carry with them for the rest of their life. Why not teach them now instead of learning in life, usually in an unpleasant way how to overcome instead of conquering and staying consistent.

Be Your Own Best Friend

One of the biggest obstacles we will have in life will be ourselves. How we talk to ourselves is detrimental to our wellbeing. In Chapter 7, I discussed how our mind can become like a recording, playing old songs that don't even apply to us, yet we keep listening to them.

Breaking a recording of speaking badly about yourself can be tough. Overcoming this means learning a whole new language of how to talk to yourself. An effective way to begin helping your child learn is to study and research together, what it means to be a friend. In learning to be a friend, a child will come to understand that it takes kindness, compassion, love, forgiveness, compromise, communication, and patience. Find books to read about being a friend. Talk about examples in both your lives about your friends. Discuss what true friendship means and what a fair-weather friend means. Not only will you be helping your child with discernment, and how to treat others, most importantly, it will circle back around to them, learning to be their own best friend.

Friendship Activity

Becoming aware of how we treat ourselves with the Friendship Activity is the first step in becoming a better friend to others and yourself. Answer the following questions with your child, in this journaling activity:

How would you want a friend to treat you?

What qualities make a good friend?

Look over the qualities that were listed and ask, is this how you treat yourself?

Go through each quality and have your child circle the ones they feel need improvement. Pick one quality, find the definition and write it down. Take time during the next week to look at that quality that needs improvement. Research, show examples, or read a book about the quality.

In what ways can you help your child learn how to become a better friend?

Forgiveness

Teaching your child at a young age the art of forgiveness can save them from years of resenting, being angry, and hurt from others. When we forgive, it doesn't excuse the behavior or hurt inflicted by another person. It releases us from the baggage of carrying around the offense of what someone else did or said to us.

Forgiveness must be practiced. Life gives us plenty of opportunities to do just that. First, we start by simply saying we forgive so and so for what happened. We may not believe it in our hearts, but the first step is saying it. Soon it will sink into us, and we will be able to let go of the offense, instead of keeping it chained to us.

THE ENVIRONMENT

What surrounds us in our environment can hold us back or help us be successful. We only have so much control with our outside environment. We can control our home environment. Help make your family's home surroundings safe with these tips:

Mold

Regularly spot checking for mold in areas that have water and piping is a necessity. Areas such as showers, drains, and under appliances can have leaks that go undetected and do costly damage to your home and health by harboring mold.

If you have mold, unhealthy symptoms it creates in the body will not go away until the mold is eradicated.

After the mold has been treated in the environment, you may also treat the body for mold toxicity. Grapefruit seed extract and activated charcoal are a few great supplements that are safe and effective to use for mold exposure. It's a good idea to keep natural mold cleaners on hand and use them regularly. In a shower, you can use tea tree essential oil or liquid grapefruit seed extract mixed with water. These are both free of chemicals, safe, non-toxic, and can be applied after each use of the shower.

Mold exposure symptoms can include fatigue, brain fog, achy muscles, chronic infections, congestion, asthma-like symptoms, arthritis-like symptoms, night sweats, tics, and tremors.

Candida

If you feel as though your child may be suffering from Candida, many natural products are safe and effective to use. Products worth buying:

Oregano- If you are using the essential oil, only use on older children.

Black Walnut- Very effect in an alcohol-free tincture.

Pau D'Arco Tea- For the best results, drink 3 small cups of tea per day. Adding peppermint, cinnamon, or another flavored herbal tea may help make this tea more appealing to your child.

Garlic-Try to include garlic, on a regular basis, in your child's diet to keep candida at bay.

Tea tree oil- Tea tree oil is safe to use topically without dilution. Add a few drops to your child's shampoo to get rid of cradle cap and keep lice away!

Probiotics- Putting good bacteria back in the body, in the form of probiotics, can help keep candida populations low.

An overgrowth of yeast can look like yellowing of nails, peeling skin, cradle cap on the head or eyebrows, areas of itchiness, redness, dandruff, rashes, yeast-like discharge, sugar cravings, leaky gut syndrome, fatigue, low thyroid, allergies, and sensitivities.

Heavy Metals

If your child has been exposed to heavy metals in any way, chelation can alleviate the symptoms. Chelation using natural means, such as foods, is safe and effective. Chelators to include in the child's diet:

Chlorella, Spirulina, Parsley, Cilantro, and Apples.

Heavy metal exposure can induce symptoms like sensitivities, allergies, brain fog, loss of concentration, confusion, chronic infections, hyperactivity, forgetfulness, and attention problems.

Clutter

The structure of the environment is more important than one may think. Many children have an abundance of toys. Having too much of anything can be overwhelming and a huge stressor. Taking the opportunity to weed out excess, with or without your child, is beneficial. Let's start by arranging your home in a way that works for your family.

Whole House Assessment

Just as you journaled an inventory of nutrition and health for your child, it is time to inventory the environment in which your child is in. Pick an area of your home, starting slowly on a timeline that works for you, dive in, and arrange your environment. With a clipboard, go room to room and assess the work that needs to be done.

When starting in a room, it is best to get four boxes or bags lined up. One for trash, one recycles, one to sell, and the last one you can donate to a friend or organization. Keep in mind the goal is to keep what you need and use. All the rest creates clutter, which is toxic to the environment.

Whole House Assessment

Look over the rooms in your house and as answer the following questions:

Kitchen/Breakfast/Dining Area

What about this room stresses you or a family member out?

Do you like the flow of the area?

Is there enough walking room?

Is there too much furniture?

What isn't working?

What is working?

Are there piles that need to be gone through?

Does everything in the room belong in the area?

Are the cabinets clearly organized?

Do you have too much in the drawers or cabinets? Are they filled to the max? Is it easy to find what you need?

Do all the lids have a mate?

Have any small appliances to donate to free up space?

Is your cookware peeling or scratched?

Is anything broken that needs to be fixed or thrown away?

Do your oven mitts work or are they too thinned or have holes?

Do you use all your cookbooks?

Are chemicals put away, out of reach of children and animals?

Is your pantry divided in categories or grouped together, so it is easy to see items such as snacks, cereals, spices, and canned foods?

Would baskets, dividers, or bins help?

Would labeling help?

Expired or outdated food eliminated?

Can you donate any unwanted, non-perishable food?

Under the sink, clean and dry? No water damage or mold present?

Additional comments:

Family Room Area-

What about this room stresses you or a family member out?

Do you like to think flow of the area?

Is there enough walking room?

Is there too much furniture?

What is working and isn't working?

Are there piles that need to be gone through?

Does everything in the room belong in the family room?

Do you have too much in the drawers or cabinets? Are they filled to the max? Is it easy to find what you need?

Would baskets, dividers, or bins help?

Would labeling help?

Are there too many toys? Do all the toys get used?

Is anything broken that needs to be fixed or thrown away?

Additional comments:

Bathrooms-

What about this room stresses you or a family member out?

What isn't working?

What is working?

Are the cabinets clearly organized?

Do you have too much in the drawers or cabinets? Are they filled to the max? Is it easy to find what you need?

Are chemicals put away, out of reach of children and animals?

Would baskets, dividers, or bins help?

Would labeling help?

Any expired or outdated products?

Under the sink, clean and dry? No mold present?

Shower clean and free from mold?

Bathtub clean and free from mold?

Are there piles to go through?

Does everything in the room belong in the bathroom?

Is anything broken that needs to be fixed or thrown away?

Additional comments:

Bedrooms-

What about this room stresses you or a family member out?

Do you like the flow of the area?

Is there enough walking room?

Is there too much furniture?

What isn't working?

What is working?

Are there drawers that need to be organized? Are they filled to the max? Is it easy to find what you need?

Would baskets, dividers, or bins help?

Would labeling help?

Are there too many knick-knacks?

Are there too many sheets, pillows or blankets?

Are there piles that need to be gone through?

Does everything belong in the bedroom?

Is anything broken that needs to be fixed or thrown away?

Additional comments:

Closets-

What about this area stresses you or a family member out?

Do you like the flow of the area?

Is there enough walking room?

What is working and isn't working?

Would baskets, dividers, or bins help?

Would labeling help?

Do you have too many clothes? Do they all fit? Have you worn them in the last year?

Do you have too many shoes? Do they all fit? Have they been worn in the last year?

Are you keeping worn out or clothes/shoes with holes?

Are you harboring things you never use in your closet? Is there excess that can be taken out?

Does everything belong in the closet?

Are there toys the kids no longer use?

Is anything broken that needs to be fixed or thrown away?

Additional comments:

Hallway-

What about this room stresses you or a family member out?

Do you like the flow of the area?

What does not work?

What does work?

Is there enough walking room?

Is there too much furniture?

Are there piles that need to be gone through?

Does everything that belongs in the hallway area?

Is there anything broken that needs to be fixed or thrown away?

Additional comments:

Garage/Shed/Outside Area

What about this room stresses you or a family member out?

Do you like to think the flow of the area?

Is there enough walking room?

Is there too much furniture?

What isn't working?

What is working?

Are there piles that need to be gone through?

Does everything in the room belong in the area?

Are you harboring things you never use in the garage? Is there excess that can be taken out?

Would baskets, dividers, or bins help?

Would labeling help?

Are there too many toys? Do all the toys get used?

Is anything broken that needs to be fixed or thrown away?

Are chemicals put away, out of reach of children and animals?

Do you have too much in the drawers, cabinets, and shelves? Are they filled to the max? Is it easy to find what you need?

Can any items be donated?

Additional comments:

Laundry Room-

What about this room stresses you or a family member out?

Do you like to think the flow of the area?

Is there enough walking room?

What isn't working?

What is working?

Are there piles that need to be gone through?

Does everything in the room belong in the area?

Are you harboring things never used in the laundry room? Is there excess that can be taken out?

Would baskets, dividers, or bins help?

Would labeling help?

Is anything broken that needs to be fixed or thrown away?

Are chemicals put away, out of reach of children and animals?

Do you have too much in drawers, cabinets, and shelves? Are they filled to the max? Is it easy to find what you need?

Can any items be donated?

Additional comments:

Well, you did it! You made it through the Program! Congratulations for all the small and big changes that YOU have created. YOU have made a lasting positive impact on your child's life and health. Take time to celebrate all that has been accomplished. And I thank you, for going on this journey with me. As parents, we must make decisions for our child that can be super tough. It's hard to know what the right thing to do is, until you step out and try it. I am so happy you trusted me and let me come into your family, to help be a guide. Together, we will make a difference in the world by starting with our family first.

Journal Points

Whole House Assessment

Final Thought

Anyone can complain and talk about wanting a change.
It takes a brave person to start, stick with and follow
through with any transformation.

CHAPTER 15

STICKING POINTS

MY CHILD FEELS DEPRIVED!

To combat your child feeling deprived, I suggest a
few things that will take extra work but will pay off in
the end when your child feels like he or she is not going
without. Anytime your child will be receiving some type
of food they won't be able to eat, send a matching food
they can eat. For example, if a teacher will be handing
out cupcakes for a class party and you know this ahead
of time, inquire about what the cupcake will look like
and try to match it. If the cupcake is chocolate and your
child doesn't like chocolate, substitute it with their
favorite kind. Instead of feeling outcasted, they will feel
special because you took the time to either make their
favorite treat or made a cupcake like everyone else's. It
may do some good to write an email to your child's
teacher or teachers at the beginning of the year
explaining the situation, asking them to let you know
ahead of time if there will be treats served.

Another thing that you can do is instead of talking
about what your child can't eat, talk about what your
child can eat. For instance, if you are at a restaurant, and
there are two items on the menu your child can eat,
focus on the two, and not the rest. Or if your child can't

have any of the beverages offered except water, ask if they would like lemon or lime in their water to flavor it. Whatever you focus on will become bigger, so if you focus on what they can't have, trouble has had an invitation!

I AM OVERWHELMED!

During this process, if you look too far ahead at where you are now and what needs to be done, it can be overwhelming. Having an end goal is a great idea. Feeling negatively about the situation because you are not meeting your goal as quickly as you would like, will not help in any way. You are where you are supposed to be. There are lessons in every single trial. The hard work you are putting in now will pay off in your family's future. When you start feeling that feeling of overwhelm, just breathe. It's going to be ok. It may not feel ok at all, but it will all happen when it is supposed to. Love yourself, be kind, and take a break.

WHAT IF I DO THIS AND NOTHING WORKS?

There will be an improvement from cleaning up your child's diet. It may take a while before you see results. Your child didn't get this way overnight and reversing the effects won't take overnight either.

NOTHING SEEMS TO BE HELPING!

If you feel like no matter what you do, nothing seems to help, or you feel something is missing, I would suggest a few things. First and foremost, never give up. Keep in mind your child will not change overnight. Keep trying; your answer is out there. Try going back and do Step 1 of the program for another week. Record everything you can about your child's habits. It may seem like a lot of work, but when you put everything together on paper, oftentimes, you discover a pattern.

If you followed the Steps in the Program completely and still see no result, it may be time for you to enlist help on a one on one basis. Check my website to see how we can work together, one on one. If you would like help in person, try finding a professional in your area in the fields of Natural Medicine or Practices. Chiropractors, Naturopathic, Functional and Integrative Doctors or Practitioners can perform proper testing for sensitivities and intolerances.

THIS IS TOO MUCH WORK!

No, too much work is dealing with your child's bad behavior!!!

WHY AM I DOING THIS?

Your child is trusting you for help. No child wants to misbehave and disappoint their parents. Invest in your children right now, so they can have the future they deserve!

PICKY EATING

Most parents have to deal with picky eating, so no worries! It just means you'll have to be a little more creative in the kitchen. Try letting your child help prepare meals and snacks. Put them in charge of encouraging other family members to try new foods. Reward them for a small bite of a new different food. If they refuse to try anything new, puree foods and sneak them into meals and snacks.

If you still have a problem with picky eating, be aware that it can be a deficiency in Zinc. Try serving foods that are high in Zinc like nuts, seeds, red meat, eggs, and potatoes. Trying a Zinc supplement at a low dose may be helpful. Other signs of zinc deficiency are white spots on the nails, pica (eating and craving inappropriate items that are nonfoods like paper or dirt), and paper-thin nails. Be aware, too much Zinc in the diet can cause diarrhea, nausea, headaches, and loss of appetite.

CRAVINGS

Cravings are a message the body is trying to send signaling something is out of balance. Do not ignore cravings! They are important and can lead you to something taking place in the body. They can guide you like a map. Cravings are a deficiency in something missing that the body wants and needs. Causes for cravings may be due to a lack of a nutrient like vitamins and minerals, a lack of emotion like feeling loved and wanted, or an overabundance of stress.

Common cravings and what might cause them:

Chocolate- Lack of magnesium.

Salt- Thyroid deficiency, sweating excessively or lack of a mineral.

Sugar- Low blood sugar, depression, loneliness, or an overgrowth of yeast.

Bread or complex carbs- Low blood sugar, lack of protein, or an overgrowth of yeast.

Hunger- Can be thirst, body not digesting and getting nourished, or emotions not being met.

WHEN ONE PARENT PARTICIPATES, AND THE OTHER DOESN'T

There is nothing more frustrating than trying to help your child meet their fundamental needs, such as the right foods, quality sleep, and practicing exercises, and the other parent doesn't agree or participate. Reading this book shows that you are plugged into your child, and you are trying to be the best parent you can be. You can choose to be consistent, no matter if the other parent is not.

Preaching health to the other parent most likely will not work. Actions speak louder than words, so lead by example. Stay consistent; keep doing right by your child.

By staying on track with your child, when they fall off their healthy routine, chances are it won't affect them as it once did. Just get back on track and start again. Do the best you can for your child and move on!

SOCIETY AND VIEWS ON FOOD

People care for others with food. People want you to enjoy the foods that they enjoy. I have been in quite a few situations of my own, where I felt the pressure of other people wanting me to eat something that I knew would bother me. Do not give in to pressure because of what someone else wants you to do. When you are in this situation, remember, who will suffer if the food is eaten? It won't be the people putting the pressure on. Try to keep in perspective; we eat to fuel our bodies. Social events may center around foods, but keep in mind, social interaction, and the connections your child makes will make the most memorable part of any event.

WHAT TO DO WHEN PEOPLE DON'T UNDERSTAND

A large majority of the general public that eats a Standard American Diet, has a hard time understanding healthy eating. I know I did before I went on my health journey. Most people think eating healthy is a diet, when it should be the way we have always eaten. Many people wait until their body is in poor condition, before they decide to eat healthier.

There will always be a part of the population that will not understand why you parent the way you choose to. Some of the hardest people that judge you, may very well be your family and friends. Since a guidebook doesn't come with children when they are born, other people will not know what is best for your child. They may think they know what is best and vocalize it to you. Remember, this child is your child. Trust your instincts as a parent and do what's best. You were given your child for a reason, and no one else has the privilege of raising them but you. Having an open mind to other suggestions is always a good idea, but never compromise what's in your heart because someone else told you to do things a certain way. Check your heart; it'll never steer you wrong. Stand firm and carry on.

BIRTHDAY PARTIES AND OTHER EVENTS

Birthday parties can be fun and exciting for your child! Parties can also be a great place to eat foods that may adversely affect your child. The best way to deal with this is not to deny your child the right to engage with their friends. Do not stop them from going or tell them if they go, they cannot eat. Being super strict can backfire with children rebelling into activities, which can play a big role in unhealthy relationships with food. It's always best to improvise and compromise.

One way to improvise is to find out the foods that will be served at the party and replace them with a healthy version. If ice cream will be served, but your child is dairy-free, bring a scoop of dairy-free ice cream.

If pizza is will be served, but your child is gluten-free, bring a gluten-free pizza for them. Doing this does take time and effort on your part, but you will thank yourself later when your child is symptom free.

A compromise for your child could be giving them a choice of what they would like to eat at the party. If hot dogs are being served, but your child is corn-free and isn't crazy about hot dogs anyway, ask your child, "would you like me to make you a hot dog, or would you like me to make you something else?" (By the way, most hot dogs do have some form of corn in the ingredients.)

Never make food a big deal for your child. The goal is smooth transitions and interactions with food. Making a big deal about food will only set them up for future problems. If they question you about why they can't eat like everyone else, it's ok to be honest. Tell them the truth; some food makes their body react badly.

VISITS WITH FAMILY AND FRIENDS WITHOUT YOU

Your child will likely have a sleepover with a friend or a family member without you. Never deprive them of having special time with friends or family because you have different ideas of health compared to them. The goal is to teach your child from a young age to be independent and make good decisions, never to deprive them of experiences because they eat a certain way. Talking to your children appropriately for their age group and being honest will always be best in the long run.

Sending food with your child is a safe, easy, and a practical answer for overnights and visits. It takes the pressure off the other adults to find appropriate foods. The child can focus on having fun and not worrying about experiencing symptoms because of something they ate. If you run into the problem of the adults not understanding, read the question, in this chapter, about when others do not understand.

FALLING OFF THE WAGON OR LETTING THINGS GO

Let me start by saying, this could very well happen. No one is perfect. There will be times things will get missed. There will be times in desperation, something will be allowed that you usually wouldn't allow. There will be times you think I should, I could, I wished I would of. I'm here to tell you; it's ok! You are ok! Your child will be ok.

Making a healthy lifestyle choice is about consistency, not perfection. Consistency will ensure that when you do fall off that wagon, it'll be easier to get back on and recover from. Don't be harsh on yourself or your child ever. Be your own best friend, just like what you teach your child. Love yourself and realize it will all be ok. Learn what you can do to improve and move on. Don't waste time on guilt, sadness, worrying, being anxious or anything else negative.

If your child eats something occasionally that is off their program, they will feel the difference. Having your child feel the difference between healthy and unhealthy is a beautiful thing! It will teach them self-control and help them stick to good decisions when you're not there to help them.

PARTNERSHIP

Feeling a bit stuck and need some additional ideas or help? If you still feel yourself struggling after you do the Steps or feel like you need a partner to walk hand in hand with you through this process, consider partnering with me to help take you to the next level.

As an Integrative Health Coach, I look at all the core areas of your child's life that influence their health and wellbeing. I focus on the needs of the family and work to individualize a program for a proper fit. I am here to listen, help, and guide you with your personal family goals. Being able to talk, trust, and feel supported during any transition can make all the difference in a successful outcome!

Visit brittahelayne.com for more information.

APPENDIX

SYMPTOMS CHECKLIST

DAILY JOURNAL

INGREDIENTS CHECKLIST

WEEKLY MENU

CREATE THE CHANGE

WHOLE HOUSE ASSESSMENT

Symptoms Checklist

Ruling out sensitivities is important and can make a huge difference in a child's behavior. If you feel like your child may have a sensitivity reaction to food, but you are not sure what the food is, taking this Symptoms Checklist can help.

Does your child have symptoms of a food sensitivity? Circle or highlight the symptoms below that you feel your child exhibits. If there are symptoms that your child has that are not on the list, write them on the lines below.

Behavior- ADD/ADHD behavior (inattentiveness, hyperactive, lack of focus, restless), OCD behaviors (obsessive and repetitive behavior), irritability, poor eye contact, food cravings, poor comprehension, anger, brain fog, aggression, lack of interest, disorganized thinking and disorientation, anxiety, depression, moodiness, over emotional, inappropriate laughter

Circulatory System- elevated blood pressure, racing heart, irregular pulse

Digestive System- upset stomach, IBS, constipation, diarrhea, mucus in stool, nausea, vomiting, gas, cramping, heartburn, bloating, abdominal pain

General- fatigue, delayed growth, delayed puberty, lethargy, speech disorders, vision problems, cravings

Neurological System- headaches, migraines, dizziness, ears ringing, tics, insomnia, night terrors, sleep disruptions

Respiratory System- coughing, sore throat, clearing throat constantly, canker sores in the mouth, bleeding or swollen gums, tooth discoloration, excess mucus, runny nose, congestion, watery or itchy eyes, sinus problems, ear infections, nasal polyps

Skeletal and Muscular System- aches and pains, swelling, stiffness

Skin- dark circles under the eyes, rosy red cheeks and ears, acne, hair loss, skin disruptions and disorders, rashes, elbow rash, eczema, hives

Urinary System- edema, bladder infections

Others:

_____
_____
_____
_____
_____
_____
_____
_____

Common Offenders That Produce Symptoms

Any Sensitivity

Aches and Pains	Heartburn
Bloating	Irregular Pulse
Coughing	Irritability
Dark Circles Under Eyes	Racing Heart
Elevated Blood Pressure	Skin Rash and Hives
Fatigue	Swelling and Stiffness
Food Cravings	Throat Clearing
	Watery Itchy Eyes

Corn

ADD/ADHD Behavior	Lack of Concentration
Aggression	Lack of Focus
Anger	Moodiness
Anxiety	Night Terrors
Behavior Problems	OCD Behavior
Brain Fog	Skin Disruption and
Headaches	Disorders
Hyperactivity	Sleep Disruptions
	Tics

Dairy/Soy/Casein

Acne	Frequent Sinus Infections
Anxiety	IBS Constipation/Diarrhea
Behavioral Issues	Inappropriate Laughter
Brain Fog	Lack of Interest
Congestion	Mucus in Stools
Depression	Poor Comprehension
Eczema	Poor Eye Contact
Excess Mucus	Repetitive Behavior
Frequent Ear	Rosy Red Cheeks or Ears
Infections	Runny Nose
	Sore Throat

Gluten

ADD/ADHD	Eczema
Behavior	Elbow Rash
Anxiety	Frequent Bladder Infections
Bleeding or Swollen	Headaches
Gums	Inappropriate Laughter
Brain Fog	Lack of Interest
Canker Sores	Nausea
Constipation	Over Emotional/Moodiness
Cramping	Poor Comprehension
Delayed Growth	Poor Eye Contact
Delayed Puberty	Repetitive Behavior
Diarrhea	Tooth Discoloration
	Vomiting

Additives- Preservatives/Dyes/Flavor Enhancers/Fragrances

Abdominal Pain	Hyperactivity
Acne	Insomnia
Aggression	Lack of Concentration
Behavior Problems	Lack of Focus
Congestion	Lethargy
Disorganized Thinking	Migraines
Disorientation	Mood Swings
Dizziness	Nasal Polyps
Ear Infection	Nausea
Eczema	Ringing in Ears
Edema	Skin Rash
Gas	Speech Disorder
Headaches	Tics
Heartburn	Upset Stomach
Hives	Vision Problems

(Please note, symptoms can vary in each individual.)

DATE:

DAILY JOURNAL

A DAY IN THE LIFE OF_____

SLEEP	EXERCISE	QUIET TIME
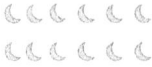	10 10 10	
	10 10 10	

Awake: Asleep:

Daily Meals and Snacks

Time   Foods   Symptoms

WATER

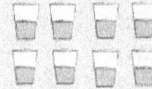

ENVIRONMENT
STRESSORS

NOTES

_____

_____

_____

_____

214

ADDITIVES

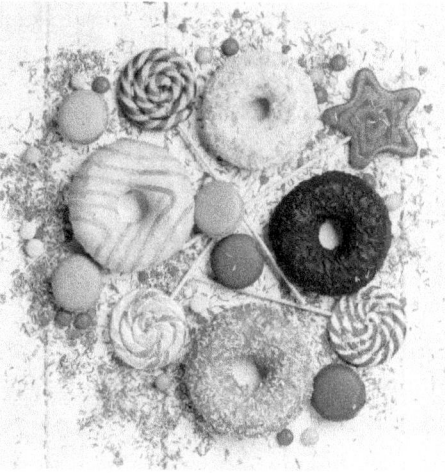

All Artificial food Coloring

All Artificial Sweeteners

BHA

BHT

BPA

Coloring

Fragrances

MSG

Nitrates

Nitrites

PFC

Perchlorate

TBHQ

If it sounds like a chemical, it probabaly is.

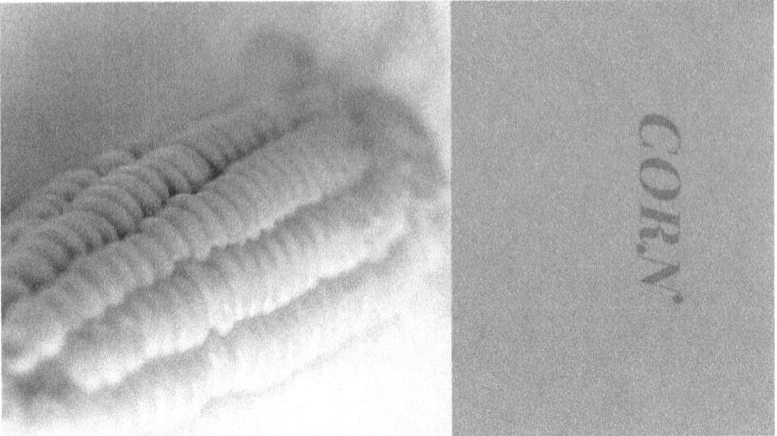

CORN

Alcohol
Artificial & Natural Flavors
Aspartame
Baking Powder
Bleached & Enriched Flour
Bleached & Enriched Sugar
Carmel & Carmel Coloring
Corn Starch
Flavoring
Food Starch
Cereal
Citric Acid
Confectioners Sugar
Anything with Corn
Crystalline Fructose
Dahlia Syrup
Dextrin & Dextrose
Erythritol
Folic Acid
Fructose
Glucose
Golden Syrup
Grits
Hominy
Hydrolyzed Protein

High Fructose Corn Syrup
Invert Sugar & Invert Syrup
Isoglucose
Lactic Acid
Lecithin
Maize
Malt
Maltitol
Maltodextrin
Mannitol
Modified Food Starch
MSG
Pectin
Polysorbate
Sorbitol
Starch
Vegetable Gum
Vinegar
Vitamin A
Vitamin C
Vitamin E
Xanthan Gum
Xylitol
Yeast
Zein

216

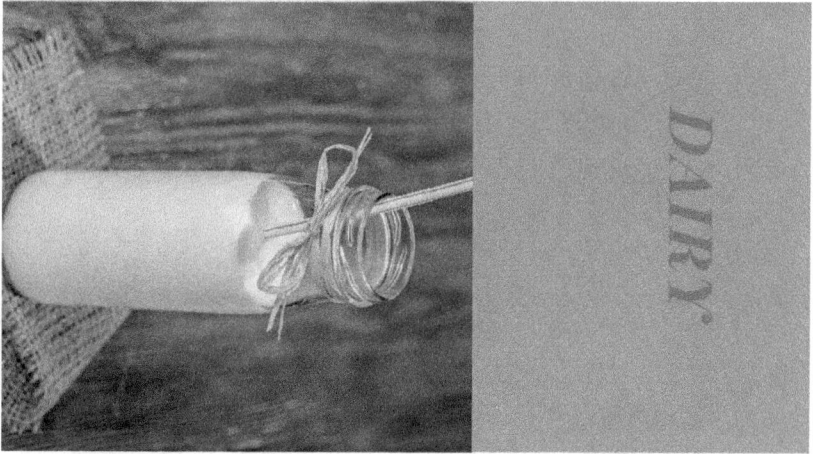

DAIRY

Artificial Butter and Flavor
Butter
Butter Extract
Buttermilk
Caesin
Caseinate
Cheese
Cheese Flavor
Condensed Milk
Cottage Cheese
Cream
Curds
Custard
Dry Milk
Evaporated Milk
Frozen Yogurt
Galactose
Ghee
Half and Half
Hydrolysates
Ice Cream
Kefir

Lactalbumin
Lactate Solids
Lactyc Yeast
Lactalbumin Phosphate
Lactoglobulin
Lactose
Lactulose
Milk
Milk Chocolate
Milk Solids
Nisin
Nougat
Pudding
Quark
Rennet
Sour Cream
Imitation Sour Cream
Whey
Whip Cream
Whipped Cream
Yogurt

217

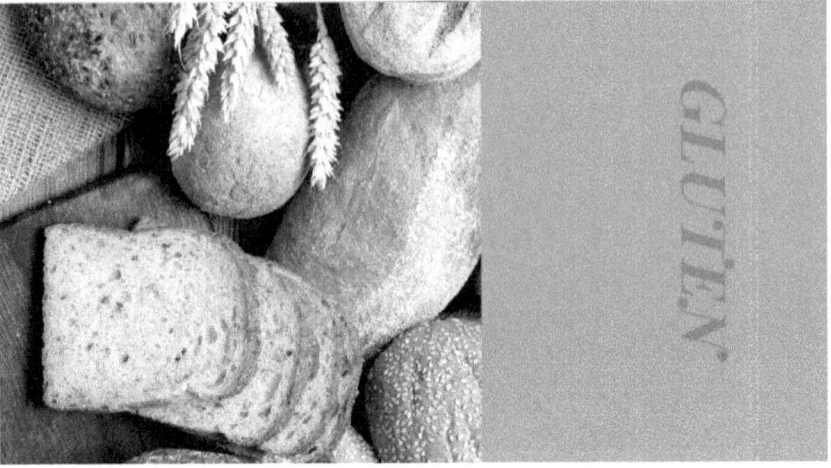

GLUTEN

All Purpose Flour
Atta
Barley
Brewer's Yeast
Bran
Bread
Bread Crumbs
Bulgar
Club Flour
Couscous
Cracker Meal
Durum
Eikorn
Emmer
Farina
Fu
Gluten
Graham Flour
Groats
Kamut
Maida
Malt
Matzo
Modified Food Starch

MSG
Natural Flavors
Noodles
Pasta
Oats
Rye
Seitan
Semolina
Spelt
Sprouted Wheat
Starch
Tabbouleh
Thickeners
Triticale
Triticum
Wheat
Wheat Berries
Wheat Bran
Wheat Germ
Wheat Grass
Wheat Protein Isolate
White Flour
Whole Meal Flour
Yeast Extract

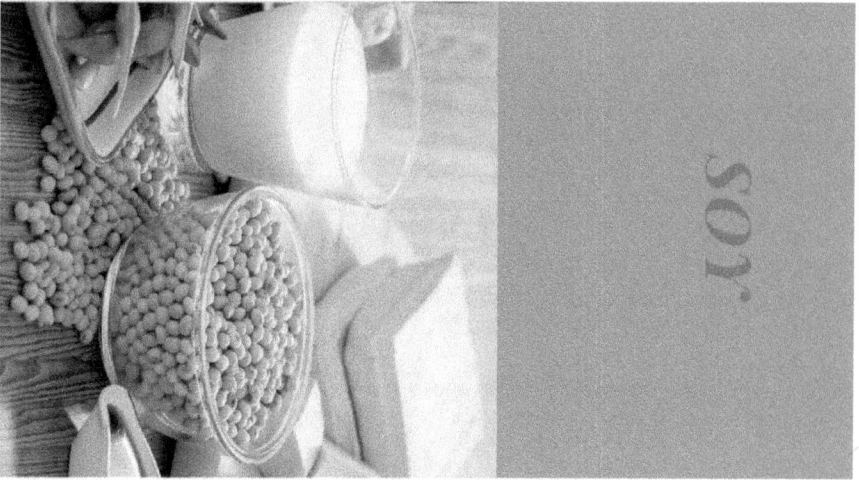

Soy

Artificial Flavors
Bean Curd
Edamame
Hydrolyzed Vegetable Protein
Kinako
Koya Dofu
Lecithin
Margarine
Mayonnaise
Miso
Mono & Diglycerides
Natto
Natural Flavors
Olean
Okara
Soy Formula
Soy Grits
Soy Lecithin
Soy Milk
Soy Miso
Soy Nuts
Soy Protein

Soy Protein Concentrate
Soy Protein Isolate
Soy Sauce
Soy Sprouts
Shoyu
Sobee
Soybean
Soybean Curds
Soybean Flour
Soybean Paste
Soya
Soya Flour
Tamari
Tempeh
Teriyaki Sauce
Tofu
Vegetable Broth
Vegetable Oil
Vegetable Shortening
Vegetable Starch
Vitamin E
Yuba

WEEKLY MENU

5-Day Meal and Snack Planner

MONDAY

BREAKFAST	Oatmeal with Wild Blueberries
LUNCH	Turkey Roll Up, Bean Chips with Salsa
DINNER	BBQ Chicken Stuffed Potato with Ranch Avocado Dip
SNACKS	Apple and Nut Butter/ Homemade Trail Mix

TUESDAY

BREAKFAST	Yogurt with Power Bites
LUNCH	Grilled Chicken Strips, Celery & Avocado Dip, Peaches
DINNER	Quesadillas
SNACKS	Crackers, Pepperoni &Cheese/Cinnamon Apples&Pecans

WEDNESDAY

BREAKFAST	Smoothie and Trail Mix
LUNCH	Lettuce Wraps, Kale Chips, Pickles and Orange Slices
DINNER	Tortilla Soup
SNACKS	Nuts and Grapes/Homemade french fries

THURSDAY

BREAKFAST	Eggs and Salsa
LUNCH	Salad with Garlic Bread
DINNER	Homemade Pizza and Pesto
SNACKS	Yogurt and Fruit/Date Rolls

FRIDAY

BREAKFAST	Banana Bread and Chicken Sausage
LUNCH	Leftover Pizza and Pineapple Rings
DINNER	Hamburgers with Roasted Sweet Potato Fries
SNACKS	Smoothie/Pretzels with Pesto

Create the Change

For each different category of health, answer the set of questions to help layout the obstacle, solution, goal, and action steps. Take your time and answer each question using details.

Example of a general answer and a detailed answer:

General response: *I would like a yard that is healthy and pretty.*

Detailed response: *I would like a tree in my yard to provide a large area of shade, shrubs that grow large enough to serve as privacy for my windows, and flowering plants placed all over to create colorful bursts of beauty.*

Examples of answers are listed for all the questions in each category. If more help is needed, refer to Chapter 14, Special Help. This activity is also in the Appendix of this book. If you would like to print the pages off, please go to my Website and go to the menu heading Tools.

Nutrition *Example*

Pick one to three different areas of nutrition you would like to see the most significant change. For each one, answer the following questions:

What would you like to change most about nutrition for your child?

I want my child to eat less starchy carbs for snacks in the form of crackers, bars, and chips and have him eat more fruits and vegetables.

I want to cook more dinners and snacks from scratch using fresh ingredients and herbs and spices.

I want to try to add more variety to my meals. I find myself using the same recipes over and over.

Which of those changes would you like to start with first, and why?

I want to start with my child eating more fruits and vegetables for snacks because I feel like this is the place where I can make the biggest impact for him to get more vitamins and minerals his growing body needs.

If you had that in place, what would the end goal look like?

Snacks would be a variety of fresh whole fruits and vegetables. My kitchen would be stocked with fresh foods instead of boxes and bags of prepared foods. Snacks will be well balanced and nutritiously dense.

After meeting the goal, how would you and your child feel? What would this mean for your family?

I would feel like my child was getting more natural nutritionally complete foods full of vitamins and minerals. My child would feel healthier, more energetic, and have a higher self-outlook about his body, eating fresh whole fruits and vegetables. Eating this way would save money on wasted produce and buying snacks that are boxed and higher priced.

What are the steps you can take to create that change?

1. I will have my child help pick out fruits and vegetables at the grocery store or a farmer's market.

2. I will make ready-made snack trays that include his selections of fresh fruit and vegetables and a starchy carb, so he has a little of what he wants while getting fresh produce.

3. I will add nutritious dips made with fresh produce and herbs, so he is eating double the amount of fresh fruits and vegetables.

Nutrition

Pick one to three different areas of nutrition you would like to see the most significant change. For each one, answer the following questions:

What would you like to change most about nutrition for your child?

Which of those changes would you like to start with first, and why?

If you had that in place, what would the end goal look like?

After meeting the goal, how would you and your child feel? What would that mean for your family?

What are the steps you can take to create that change?

Physical Fitness *Example*

Pick one to three different areas of physical fitness, you would like to see the most significant change. For each one, answer the following questions:

What would you like to change most about physical fitness for your child?

My children spend too much time playing on their phones and not enough time being physically active.

I want my children to take more of an interest in exercising to help them stay fit, flexible, and injury-free.

Which of those changes would you like to start with first, and why?

I want my children to take more interest in physical fitness in their life so they will have healthier bodies.

If you had that in place, what would the end goal look like?

My children would be getting at least 60 minutes thorough out the day of exercise. They would be physically fit, ready to take on adventures such as hiking, camping, or other activities that require endurance that they would like to try and not have to worry about injuries, lack of health, incoordination.

After meeting the goal, how would you and your child feel? What would this mean for your family?

My child would feel strong, capable, and more confident, knowing they have strength and endurance. We could do activities together that would create opportunities to bond with one another.

What are the steps you can take to create that change?

1. Together, we will choose an activity the whole family can participate in as a goal, such as hiking on a 5-mile trail. We will research places hike and decide when and where to go on our family outing.

2. We will determine what exercises to do, to get in shape for a hike and how often to exercise.

3. I will make a chart to list out the exercises; each of us can post and follow.

4. We will each do those exercises for a reasonable amount of time weekly.

5. On the decided date, we will go on the 5-mile hike.

Physical Fitness

Pick one to three different areas of physical fitness you would like to see the most significant change. For each one, answer the following questions:

What would you like to change most about physical fitness for your child?

Which of those changes would you like to start with first, and why?

If you had that in place, what would the end goal look like?

After meeting the goal, how would you and your child feel? What would that mean for your family?

What are the steps you can take to create that change?

Sleep and Meditation *Example*

What would you like to change most about sleep and meditation for your child?

I have a teenager that stays up too late at night and is not getting the amount of sleep his body needs. The lack of sleep is affecting his moods and his performance in school.

I want to help my child learn a meditation, but I don't know how to begin.

My children have no set bedtime routine. Some nights they are up until midnight. My husband and I are always tired the next day. We can't seem to get a handle on the problem.

Which of those changes would you like to start with first, and why?

I want to teach my child to meditate, so when he gets upset, he will have something to help him calm himself immediately.

If you had that in place, what would the end goal look like?

My child would be able to control his emotions and catch himself before he gets out of control. Ultimately, he will be able to feel himself when he starts to get upset and know what to do to calm down.

After meeting the goal, how would you and your child feel? What would that mean for your family?

My child would feel less stressed out and overwhelmed and be able to handle tough situations in a better way.

I would feel relieved and happy that I was able to teach something my child can carry into the future. Together, we could all learn the skills to become more peaceful individuals, which will positively affect our family dynamics.

What are the steps you can take to create that change?

1. Research and choose a few meditations that I would like to try with my child.

2. I will ask my child which meditation he would like to try.

3. I will create a special meditation corner that any family member can go to if they are feeling upset, stressed, or out of control.

4. My child and I will decorate the corner. We will put a few snacks, water bottles, books, a soft blanket, and a pillow in the area.

5. We will practice the specific meditation, and I will make a laminated sheet to follow as a guide.

Sleep and Meditation

Pick one to three different areas of sleep and meditation you would like to see the most significant change. For each one, answer the following questions:

What would you like to change most about sleep and meditation for your child?

Which of those changes would you like to start with first, and why?

If you had that in place, what would the end goal look like?

After meeting the goal, how would you and your child feel? What would that mean for your family?

What are the steps you can take to create that change?

The Mind *Example*

What would you like to change most about the mind for your child?

My child has low self-confidence. She won't try anything new because she feels as though she won't be able to do the activity.

My child keeps saying he is stupid and not good at reading.

My child is hanging around friends that aren't the best influence. I feel like this is because he has a low self-outlook about himself.

Which of those changes would you like to start with first, and why?

I want to help my child stop saying he's stupid and not good at reading. I don't want him to grow up thinking he can't learn. Thinking this way, gives him a negative outlook about himself.

If you had that in place, what would the end goal look like?

He would feel confident when reading and be able to read and comprehend the information. He would have a favorable view about himself.

How would you and your child feel after the goal was met? What would that mean for your family?

My child would have more confidence in himself and his schoolwork. He would be a friend to himself, thinking thoughts such as I can do anything, I put my mind to.

What are the steps you can take to create that change?

1. *Today, we will sit down and talk to see what he is interested in reading. I will assure him; reading involves practicing and I'll use an example of another time in his life that required practice.*

2. *Buy or print off stories or articles that my child might like to read.*

3. *Read to him, take turns reading, or have him read, without making him feel pressured to perform.*

4. *I will commit to a time to read with him. Practice reading with him at least 10 minutes a day 3-5 times a week.*

The Mind

Pick one to three different areas of the mind you would like to see the most significant change. For each one, answer the following questions:

What would you like to change most about the mind for your child?

Which of those changes would you like to start with first, and why?

If you had that in place, what would the end goal look like?

After meeting the goal, how would you and your child feel? What would that mean for your family?

What are the steps you can take to create that change?

The Environment *Example*

What would you like to change most about the environment for your child?

I use store-bought cleaners with chemicals, and I would like to learn how to make my own to save money and create a less toxic environment for my family.

My child's room is a mess. I would like to have an organization system in place.

The refrigerator in the kitchen needs to be cleaned out. It is always hard to find anything in it.

My house is a mess, and every room seems unorganized and cluttered.

Which of those changes would you like to start with first, and why?

I want to clean the whole house. It's cluttered, unorganized, and just a mess. Every time I look around, I get discouraged.

If you had that in place, what would the end goal look like?

Each room in the house would have a great feel to it. I would be able to get other work done and spend time with the family, instead of continually trying to clean up little messes made days ago. Everything would have a place in our home.

After meeting the goal, how would you and your child feel? What would that mean for your family?

My family and I would be proud to have an organized home. We could concentrate on everyday living and not get stressed with an unorganized house. After clearing out the clutter and putting items where they belong, we wouldn't waste so much time looking for things we misplace.

What are the steps you can take to create that change?

1. Decide on one area or room to start organizing.

2. Get four boxes, one for trash, one for donating, one to give away, and one for a future yard sale.

3. Commit to at least 30 minutes per day of work, until the room is organized.

4. *Assign family members to a task in each room.*

The Environment

Pick one to three different areas of the environment you would like to see the most significant change. For each one, answer the following questions:

What would you like to change most about the environment for your child?

Which of those changes would you like to start with first, and why?

If you had that in place, what would the end goal look like?

After meeting the goal, how would you and your child feel? What would that mean for your family?

What are the steps you can take to create that change?

Whole House Assessment

Look over the rooms in your house and as answer the following questions:

Kitchen/Breakfast/Dining Area

What about this room stresses you or a family member out?

Do you like the flow of the area?

Is there enough walking room?

Is there too much furniture?

What isn't working?

What is working?

Are there piles that need to be gone through?

Does everything in the room belong in the area?

Are the cabinets clearly organized?

Do you have too much in the drawers or cabinets? Are they filled to the max? Is it easy to find what you need?

Do all the lids have a mate?

Have any small appliances to donate to free up space?

Is your cookware peeling or scratched?

Is anything broken that needs to be fixed or thrown away?

Do your oven mitts work or are they too thinned or have holes?

Do you use all your cookbooks?

Are chemicals put away, out of reach of children and animals?

Is your pantry divided in categories or grouped together, so it is easy to see items such as snacks, cereals, spices, and canned foods?

Would baskets, dividers, or bins help?

Would labeling help?

Expired or outdated food eliminated?

Can you donate any unwanted, non-perishable food?

Under the sink, clean and dry? No water damage or mold present?

Additional comments:

Family Room Area-

What about this room stresses you or a family member out?

Do you like to think flow of the area?

Is there enough walking room?

Is there too much furniture?

What is working and isn't working?

Are there piles that need to be gone through?

Does everything in the room belong in the family room?

Do you have too much in the drawers or cabinets? Are they filled to the max? Is it easy to find what you need?

Would baskets, dividers, or bins help?

Would labeling help?

Are there too many toys? Do all the toys get used?

Is anything broken that needs to be fixed or thrown away?

Additional comments:

Bathrooms-

What about this room stresses you or a family member out?

What isn't working?

What is working?

Are the cabinets clearly organized?

Do you have too much in the drawers or cabinets? Are they filled to the max? Is it easy to find what you need?

Are chemicals put away, out of reach of children and animals?

Would baskets, dividers, or bins help?

Would labeling help?

Any expired or outdated products?

Under the sink, clean and dry? No mold present?

Shower clean and free from mold?

Bathtub clean and free from mold?

Are there piles to go through?

Does everything in the room belong in the bathroom?

Is anything broken that needs to be fixed or thrown away?

Additional comments:

Bedrooms-

What about this room stresses you or a family member out?

Do you like the flow of the area?

Is there enough walking room?

Is there too much furniture?

What isn't working?

What is working?

Are there drawers that need to be organized? Are they filled to the max? Is it easy to find what you need?

Would baskets, dividers, or bins help?

Would labeling help?

Are there too many knick-knacks?

Are there too many sheets, pillows or blankets?

Are there piles that need to be gone through?

Does everything belong in the bedroom?

Is anything broken that needs to be fixed or thrown away?

Additional comments:

Closets-

What about this area stresses you or a family member out?

Do you like the flow of the area?

Is there enough walking room?

What is working and isn't working?

Would baskets, dividers, or bins help?

Would labeling help?

Do you have too many clothes? Do they all fit? Have you worn them in the last year?

Do you have too many shoes? Do they all fit? Have they been worn in the last year?

Are you keeping worn out or clothes/shoes with holes?

Are you harboring things you never use in your closet? Is there excess that can be taken out?

Does everything belong in the closet?

Are there toys the kids no longer use?

Is anything broken that needs to be fixed or thrown away?

Additional comments:

Hallway-

What about this room stresses you or a family member out?

Do you like the flow of the area?

What does not work?

What does work?

Is there enough walking room?

Is there too much furniture?

Are there piles that need to be gone through?

Does everything that belongs in the hallway area?

Is there anything broken that needs to be fixed or thrown away?

Additional comments:

Garage/Shed/Outside Area

What about this room stresses you or a family member out?

Do you like to think the flow of the area?

Is there enough walking room?

Is there too much furniture?

What isn't working?

What is working?

Are there piles that need to be gone through?

Does everything in the room belong in the area?

Are you harboring things you never use in the garage? Is there excess that can be taken out?

Would baskets, dividers, or bins help?

Would labeling help?

Are there too many toys? Do all the toys get used?

Is anything broken that needs to be fixed or thrown away?

Are chemicals put away, out of reach of children and animals?

Do you have too much in the drawers, cabinets, and shelves? Are they filled to the max? Is it easy to find what you need?

Can any items be donated?

Additional comments:

Laundry Room–

What about this room stresses you or a family member out?

Do you like to think the flow of the area?

Is there enough walking room?

What isn't working?

What is working?

Are there piles that need to be gone through?

Does everything in the room belong in the area?

Are you harboring things never used in the laundry room? Is there excess that can be taken out?

Would baskets, dividers, or bins help?

Would labeling help?

Is anything broken that needs to be fixed or thrown away?

Are chemicals put away, out of reach of children and animals?

Do you have too much in drawers, cabinets, and shelves? Are they filled to the max? Is it easy to find what you need?

Can any items be donated?

Additional comments:

BIBLIOGRAPHY

CHAPTER 3

Introduction. (n.d.). Retrieved August 2019, from https://health.gov/dietaryguidelines/2015/guidelines/introducti on/nutrition-and-health-are-closely-related/#table-i-1.

CHAPTER 4

Balch, P. A. (2010). *Prescription for nutritional healing, fifth edition - a practical a-to-z re* (5th ed.) (pp 371,513). Penguin Books Australia.

Ballentine, Rudolph. *Diet & Nutrition: a Holistic Approach* (pp 46, 47, 49) Himalayan International Institute, 2004.

Compart, P. J., & Laake, D. (2013). *The Adhd and autism nutritional supplement handbook: the cutting-edge biomedical approach to treating the underlying deficiencies and symptoms of Adhd and autism (pp 23-25)*. Gloucester, MA: Fair Winds.

Environmental Working Group. (2019, March 20). EWG's 2019 Shopper's Guide to Pesticides in Produce™. Retrieved September 2019, from https://www.ewg.org/foodnews/summary.php.

Hoffer, Abram, et al. *Putting It All Together: The New Orthomolecular Nutrition*. (pp72-77) Keats, 1996.

Hyman, Mark. *The Blood Sugar Solution: the UltraHealthy Program for Losing Weight, Preventing Disease, and Feeling Great Now!* (pp201-203). Little, Brown and Company, 2012.

Lepore, Donald. *The Ultimate Healing System: The Illustrated Guide to Muscle Testing & Nutrition*.

(pp 11) Woodland Pub., 1998.

Levy, J. (2017, March 26). Macronutrients You Need & Top Macro Food Sources. Retrieved October 2019, from https://draxe.com/nutrition/macronutrients/.

Lipski, Elizabeth, and Mark Hyman. *Digestion Connection Exclusive Expanded Edition*. (pp41-43) Rodale, 2013.

Mercola, Joseph. (2017, September). 12 Signs You Should Drink More Water Right Now. Retrieved June 2019, from https://articles.mercola.com/sites/articles/archive/2017/09/28/dehydration-affects-brain-function.aspx.

The Gluten-Free Diet: Facts and Myths. (2019, July). Retrieved from https://gluten.org/resources/getting-started/the-gluten-free-diet-facts-and-myths/.

Types of Legumes. (n.d.). Retrieved November 2019, from https://www.glnc.org.au/legumes/types-of-legumes/.

Walia, A. (2018, March 13). Ten Scientific Studies Prove that Genetically Modified Food Can Be Harmful To Human Health. Retrieved August 2019, from https://www.globalresearch.ca/ten-scientific-studies-proving-gmos-can-be-harmful-to-human-health/5377054.

Whole Grains A to Z. (n.d.). Retrieved November 2019, from https://wholegrainscouncil.org/whole-grains-101/whole-grains-z.

CHAPTER 5

HHS Office, & Council on Sports. (2019, February 1). Physical Activity Guidelines for Americans. Retrieved September 2019, from https://www.hhs.gov/fitness/be-active/physical-activity-guidelines-for-americans/index.html.

CHAPTER 6

Amen, D. G. (2000). *Change your brain, change your life: the breakthrough program for conquering anxiety, depression, obsessiveness, anger, and impulsiveness* (pp. 99-104). New York, NY: Three River Press.

Bloom, D. (2016, November 8). Instead of detention, these students get meditation. Retrieved from https://www.cnn.com/2016/11/04/health/meditation-in-schools-baltimore/index.html.

Gaines, J. (2016, September 22). A school replaced detention with meditation. The results are stunning. Retrieved August 2019, from https://www.upworthy.com/this-school-replaced-detention-with-meditation-the-results-are-stunning.

How Much Sleep Do We Really Need? (n.d.). Retrieved July 2019, from https://www.sleepfoundation.org/articles/how-much-sleep-do-we-really-need.

Sargent, A. C. (1999). *The Other Mind's Eye: the gateway to the hidden treasures of your mind (pp. 10-15)*. Malibu, CA: Success Design International Publications.

CHAPTER 14

Pedersen, M. (2010). *Nutritional herbology: a reference guide to herbs (pp 94-96 & 163)*. Warsaw, IN: Whitman Publications.

ABOUT THE AUTHOR

Britta Helayne is a Certified Integrative Health Coach, Internationally Certified Reflexologist, and Aromatherapist that has been dedicated to Holistic Health Practices since 2007.

Being the mother of a child with past behavior problems, Britta understands the challenges parents face in today's world. In 2009, she came to a crossroads in life, trying to find answers for her son's bad behavior. At the same time, Britta was experiencing a health crisis of her own. What she learned from being sick and tired of being sick and tired, led her to transform her son, Braeden's life. Braeden was masked behind bad behaviors, and the cause was right in front of her. Britta couldn't see the answer until she took her own health journey. What she learned has inspired her to help other parents experience the same breakthroughs with their children.

Britta lives in Tucson, Arizona, surrounded by her children, family, and animals. She has four boys she adores named Cameron, Jensen, Benji, and Braeden.

www.ingramcontent.com/pod-product-compliance
Lightning Source LLC
LaVergne TN
LVHW051226080426
835513LV00016B/1441